UNIVERSITY OF MAINE
AT AUGUSTA

UNIVERSITY OF MAINE
1865

AUGUSTA, MAINE

The Effectiveness
of Social Interventions
for Homeless
Substance Abusers

The *Journal of Addictive Diseases* series:*
(formerly *Advances in Alcohol & Substance Abuse* series)

- *Behavioral and Biochemical Issues in Substance Abuse**
- *Cocaine, AIDS, and Intravenous Drug Use**
- *What Works in Drug Abuse Epidemiology**
- *Cocaine: Physiological and Physiopathological Effects**
- *Comorbidity of Addictive and Psychiatric Disorders**
- *Experimental Therapeutics in Addiction Medicine**
- *The Effectiveness of Social Interventions for Homeless Substance Abusers**
- *Recent Advances in the Biology of Alcoholism*
- *The Effects of Maternal Alcohol and Drug Abuse on the Newborn*
- *Evaluation of Drug Treatment Programs*
- *Current Controversies in Alcoholism*
- *Federal Priorities in Funding Alcohol and Drug Abuse Programs*
- *Psychosocial Constructs of Alcoholism and Substance Abuse*
- *The Addictive Behaviors*
- *Conceptual Issues in Alcoholism and Substance Abuse*
- *Dual Addiction: Pharmacological Issues in the Treatment of Concomitant Alcoholism and Drug Abuse*
- *Cultural and Sociological Aspects of Alcoholism and Substance Abuse*
- *Alcohol and Drug Abuse in the Affluent*
- *Alcohol and Substance Abuse in Adolescence*
- *Controversies in Alcoholism and Substance Abuse*
- *Alcohol and Substance Abuse in Women and Children*
- *Cocaine: Pharmacology, Addiction, and Therapy*
- *Children of Alcoholics*
- *Pharmacological Issues in Alcohol and Substance Abuse*
- *AIDS and Substance Abuse*
- *Alcohol Research from Bench to Bedside*
- *Addiction Potential of Abused Drugs and Drug Classes*

The Effectiveness of Social Interventions for Homeless Substance Abusers

Gerald J. Stahler, PhD
Guest Editor

Barry Stimmel, MD
Editor

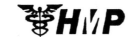

The Haworth Medical Press
An Imprint of
The Haworth Press, Inc.
New York • London

Published by

The Haworth Medical Press, 10 Alice Street, Binghamton, NY 13904-1580 USA

The Haworth Medical Press is an imprint of The Haworth Press, Inc., 10 Alice Street, Binghamton, NY 13904-1580 USA.

The Effectiveness of Social Interventions for Homeless Substance Abusers has also been published as *Journal of Addictive Diseases*, Volume 14, Number 4 1995.

The development, preparation, and publication of this work has been undertaken with great care. However, the publisher, employees, editors, and agents of The Haworth Press and all imprints of The Haworth Press, Inc., including The Haworth Medical Press and Pharmaceutical Products Press, are not responsible for any errors contained herein or for consequences that may ensue from use of materials or information contained in this work. Opinions expressed by the author(s) are not necessarily those of The Haworth Press, Inc.

Library of Congress Cataloging-in-Publication Data

The effectiveness of social interventions for homeless substance abusers / Gerald J. Stahler, guest editor [and] Barry Stimmel, editor.
    p. cm.
    Includes bibliographical references and index.
    ISBN 1-56024-807-6 (alk. paper)
    1. Homeless persons–Drug use. 2. Homeless persons–Alcohol use. 3. Narcotic addicts–Rehabilitation. 4. Alcoholics–Rehabilitation. I. Stahler, Gerald. II. Stimmel, Barry, 1939- .
HV5824.H65E35 1996   95-50799
362.29'08'6942–dc20   CIP

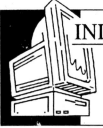

INDEXING & ABSTRACTING

Contributions to this publication are selectively indexed or abstracted in print, electronic, online, or CD-ROM version(s) of the reference tools and information services listed below. This list is current as of the copyright date of this publication. See the end of this section for additional notes.

- *Abstracts in Anthropology,* Baywood Publishing Company, 26 Austin Avenue, P.O. Box 337, Amityville, NY 11701

- *Abstracts of Research in Pastoral Care & Counseling,* Loyola College, 7135 Minstrel Way, Suite 101, Columbia, MD 21045

- *Academic Abstracts/CD-ROM,* EBSCO Publishing, P.O. Box 2250, Peabody, MA 01960-7250

- *ADDICTION ABSTRACTS,* National Addiction Centre, 4 Windsor Walk, London SE5 8AF, England

- *ALCONLINE Database,* Swedish Council for Information on Alcohol and Other Drugs, Box 27302, S-102 54 Stockholm, Sweden

- *Biosciences Information Service of Biological Abstracts (BIOSIS),* Biosciences Information Service, 2100 Arch Street, Philadelphia, PA 19103-1399

- *Brown University Digest of Addiction Theory and Application, The (DATA Newsletter),* Project Cork Institute, Dartmouth Medical School, 14 South Main Street, Suite 2F, Hanover, NH 03755-2015

- *Cambridge Scientific Abstracts, Health & Safety Science Abstracts,* Cambridge Information Group, 7200 Wisconsin Avenue #601, Bethesda, MD 20814

- *Child Development Abstracts & Bibliography,* University of Kansas, 2 Bailey Hall, Lawrence, KS 66045

- *CNPIEC Reference Guide: Chinese National Directory of Foreign Periodicals,* P.O. Box 88, Beijing, Peoples Republic of China

- *Criminal Justice Abstracts,* Willow Tree Press, 15 Washington Street, 4th Floor, Newark, NJ 07102

- *Criminal Justice Periodical Index,* University Microfilms, Inc., 300 North Zeeb Road, Ann Arbor, MI 48106

(continued)

- *Criminology, Penology and Police Science Abstracts,* Kugler Publications, P.O. Box 11188, 1001 GD Amsterdam, The Netherlands

- *Current Contents: Clinical Medicine/Life Sciences (CC: CM/LS) (weekly Table of Contents Service),* and *Social Science Citation Index.* Articles also searchable through *Social SciSearch,* ISI's online database and in ISI's *Research Alert* current awareness service. Institute for Scientific Information, 3501 Market Street, Philadelphia, PA 19104-3302

- *Educational Administration Abstracts (EAA),* Sage Publications, Inc., 2455 Teller Road, Newbury Park, CA 91320

- *Excerpta Medica/Secondary Publishing Division,* Elsevier Science Inc., Secondary Publishing Division, 655 Avenue of the Americas, New York, NY 10010

- *Health Source: Indexing & Abstracting of 160 selected health related journals, updated monthly,* EBSCO Publishing, 83 Pine Street, Peabody, MA 01960

- *Health Source Plus: expanded version of "Health Source" to be released shortly:* EBSCO Publishing, 83 Pine Street, Peabody, MA 01960

- *Index Medicus/MEDLINE,* National Library of Medicine, 8600 Rockville Pike, Bethesda, MD 20894

- *Index to Periodical Articles Related to Law,* University of Texas, 727 East 26th Street, Austin, TX 78705

- *International Pharmaceutical Abstracts,* American Society of Hospital Pharmacists, 7272 Wisconsin Avenue, Bethesda, MD 20814

- *INTERNET ACCESS (& additional networks) Bulletin Board for Libraries ("BUBL"), coverage of information resources on INTERNET, JANET, and other networks.*
  - JANET X.29: UK.AC.BATH.BUBL or 00006012101300
  - TELNET: BUBL.BATH.AC.UK or 138.38.32.45 login 'bubl'
  - Gopher: BUBL.BATH.AC.UK (138.32.32.45). Port 7070
  - World Wide Web: http: / / www.bubl.bath.ac.uk./BUBL/ home.html
  - NISSWAIS: telnetniss.ac.uk (for the NISS gateway)
  The Andersonian Library, Curran Building, 101 St. James Road, Glasgow G4 0NS, Scotland

- *Inventory of Marriage and Family Literature (online and hard copy),* Peters Technology Transfer, 306 East Baltimore Pk, 2nd Floor, Media, PA 19063

(continued)

- *Medication Use STudies (MUST) Database,* The University of Mississippi, School of Pharmacy, University, MS 38677

- *Mental Health Abstracts (online through DIALOG),* IFI/Plenum Data Company, 3202 Kirkwood Highway, Wilmington, DE 19808

- *NIAAA Alcohol and Alcohol Problems Science Database (ETOH),* National Institute on Alcohol Abuse and Alcoholism, 1400 Eye Street NW, Suite 600, Washington, DC 20005

- *PASCAL International Bibliography T205: Sciences de l'information Documentation,* INIST/CNRS-Service Gestion des Documents Primaires, 2 allee du Parc de Brabois, F-54514 Vandoeuvre-les-Nancy, Cedex, France

- *Psychological Abstracts (PsycINFO),* American Psychological Association, P.O. Box 91600, Washington, DC 20090-1600

- *Sage Family Studies Abstracts (SFSA),* Sage Publications, Inc., 2455 Teller Road, Newbury Park, CA 91320

- *Sage Urban Studies Abstracts (SUSA),* Sage Publications, Inc., 2455 Teller Road, Newbury Park, CA 91320

- *SilverPlatter Information, Inc. "CD-ROM/online,"* Information Resources Group, P.O. Box 50550, Pasadena, CA 91115-0550

- *Social Planning/Policy & Development Abstracts (SOPODA),* Sociological Abstracts, Inc., P.O. Box 22206, San Diego, CA 92192-0206

- *Social Work Abstracts,* National Association of Social Workers, 750 First Street NW, 8th Floor, Washington, DC 20002

- *Sociological Abstracts (SA),* Sociological Abstracts, Inc., P.O. Box 22206, San Diego, CA 92192-0206

- *SOMED (social medicine) Database,* Institute fur Dokumentation, Postfach 20 10 12, D-33548 Bielefeld, Germany

- *Studies on Women Abstracts,* Carfax Publishing Company, P.O. Box 25, Abingdon, Oxfordshire, OX14 3UE, United Kingdom

- *Violence and Abuse Abstracts: A Review of Current Literature on Interpersonal Violence (VAA),* Sage Publications, Inc., 2455 Teller Road, Newbury Park, CA 91320

(continued)

SPECIAL BIBLIOGRAPHIC NOTES

related to special journal issues (separates)
and indexing/abstracting

- ☐ indexing/abstracting services in this list will also cover material in any "separate" that is co-published simultaneously with Haworth's special thematic journal issue or DocuSerial. Indexing/abstracting usually covers material at the article/chapter level.

- ☐ monographic co-editions are intended for either non-subscribers or libraries which intend to purchase a second copy for their circulating collections.

- ☐ monographic co-editions are reported to all jobbers/wholesalers/approval plans. The source journal is listed as the "series" to assist the prevention of duplicate purchasing in the same manner utilized for books-in-series.

- ☐ to facilitate user/access services all indexing/abstracting services are encouraged to utilize the co-indexing entry note indicated at the bottom of the first page of each article/chapter/contribution.

- ☐ this is intended to assist a library user of any reference tool (whether print, electronic, online, or CD-ROM) to locate the monographic version if the library has purchased this version but not a subscription to the source journal.

- ☐ individual articles/chapters in any Haworth publication are also available through the Haworth Document Delivery Services (HDDS).

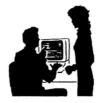

The Effectiveness of Social Interventions for Homeless Substance Abusers

CONTENTS

ABOUT THE GUEST EDITOR

Gerald Stahler, PhD, a clinical psychologist, is Associate Professor in the Department of Geography and Urban Studies at Temple University. His research interests focus on developing and evaluating social interventions for such urban problems as substance abuse, homelessness, and adolescent pregnancy. Dr. Stahler has published numerous articles in the areas of program evaluation, substance abuse, and teenage pregnancy, and recently guest co-edited an issue of *Contemporary Drug Problems* devoted to qualitative research findings concerning substance abuse treatment for homeless substance abusers. He is also the co-editor of the book *Innovative Approaches to Mental Health Evaluation* published by Academic Press. He has been a recipient of a number of research grants, and is currently studying how to successfully re-integrate homeless crack addicted women and their children back into the community using the African-American Church community. Dr. Stahler previously served as Associate Vice Provost for Research at Temple University, Director of Evaluation Research at the National Center for Family Studies at Catholic University, Vice President of Research for the Horizon Institute, a research consulting firm, and as a private practice clinician.

EDITORIAL

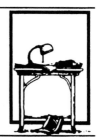

Social Interventions
for Homeless Substance Abusers:
Evaluating Treatment Outcomes

Epidemiological studies have shown that substance abuse among the homeless is far more prevalent than among the general population, although there is considerable variability in prevalence depending on the region, city, and subpopulation studied.[1-3] One recent meta-analysis of epidemiological studies found a median prevalence rate for Axis I substance use disorders among the homeless population of approximately 50

The author wishes to acknowledge the helpful comments of Eric Cohen and Joseph DuCette in the preparation of this manuscript.

[Haworth co-indexing entry note]: "Social Interventions for Homeless Substance Abusers: Evaluating Treatment Outcomes." Stahler, Gerald J. Co-published simultaneously in the *Journal of Addictive Diseases* (The Haworth Medical Press, an imprint of The Haworth Press, Inc.) Vol. 14, No. 4, 1995, pp. xv-xxvi; and: *The Effectiveness of Social Interventions for Homeless Substance Abusers* (ed: Gerald J. Stahler) The Haworth Medical Press, an imprint of The Haworth Press, Inc., 1995, pp. xiii-xxiv. Single or multiple copies of this article are available from The Haworth Document Delivery Service [1-800-342-9678; 9:00 a.m. - 5:00 p.m. (EST)].

percent.[3] Other studies have found that in certain cities crack cocaine has become particularly prevalent among homeless populations.[4-8] Despite the fact that the Institute of Medicine concluded that substance abuse represented the most predominant public health problem for people who are homeless,[9] there has been little empirical research assessing what types of treatment were effective with homeless persons.

While there is no single characteristic that distinguishes the homeless from other people (other than their lacking a permanent residence), they do represent a special challenge to substance abuse treatment providers because of their residential instability; poor economic and employment status; and their social disaffiliation in lacking personal supports and linkages with family, friends, and community institutions.[10] In many cases they are difficult to treat because they have problems in establishing relationships with treatment providers, are extremely mobile (which can preclude continuity of care), present a multiplicity of needs, often have co-existing mental disorders, and are frequently viewed by service providers as not being "desirable" or "good" patients.[11]

Because of these issues and the paucity of empirical knowledge about how to develop treatment strategies tailored to these populations, the National Institute of Alcohol Abuse and Alcoholism (NIAAA), in consultation with the National Institute on Drug Abuse (NIDA), developed a $48 million three year funding program to support the development and assessment of various treatment strategies for homeless persons with alcohol and other drug problems. Thus far, this has been the largest effort yet undertaken to develop and study substance abuse treatment effectiveness for homeless persons. Entitled Cooperative Agreements for Research Demonstration Projects on Alcohol and Other Drug Abuse Treatment for Homeless Persons, the program was authorized by the Stewart B. McKinney Homeless Assistance Act which provided funding for a variety of other housing, health, and social programs to assist homeless persons.

This book presents research from ten of the fourteen projects (note 1) funded under this NIAAA and NIDA initiative, and is the first volume devoted exclusively to reporting the results of rigorous research concerning substance abuse treatment outcomes for homeless persons (note 2).

BACKGROUND

The McKinney Act of 1987 and its subsequent amendments provided funding for two NIAAA/NIDA research demonstration programs. The first program, the Community Demonstration Grants Projects for Alcohol and Drug Abuse Treatment for Homeless Individuals (referred to as the

Round I demonstration program), funded nine projects in 1988 to develop outreach and treatment services for homeless substance abusers. The emphasis of this effort was to explore the usefulness of diverse treatment models for this population since there had been little empirical knowledge about how to develop and implement treatment models for homeless substance abusers.

In September 1990, NIAAA/NIDA made a second round of three year awards to 14 projects in different geographic locations with varying target populations and intervention strategies. The focus of this cooperative agreement program, which is the source of the present papers, was to *rigorously* assess the effectiveness of various extended interventions for homeless persons with alcohol and/or other drug problems. This program was more focused on scientific evaluation of the effectiveness of services than was the prior round, with specific requirements for certain design and measurement procedures.

All the projects described in this issue, for example, had the following design and measurement features:

- true experimental designs with random assignment of clients to subject groups.
- a core set of instruments including the Addiction Severity Index (ASI),[12] the Alcohol Dependence Scale (ADS),[13] and the housing section of the Personal History Form (PHF).[14] Most of the data presented in this issue are from the ASI.
- assessment of study participants at a minimum at intake, following discharge from treatment, and six months post-discharge. Some of the investigators collected more frequent follow-up data.
- large sample sizes varying from 149 to 722.
- high degree of follow-up, especially for this population, with all projects (except one) reporting follow-up rates of 74% or better.

What does vary considerably across studies are the geographic locations, recruitment sites (e.g., shelters, drug treatment program, other social programs), composition of the targeted homeless subpopulations (e.g., women with children, dual diagnosis, major drug of abuse), type of intervention implemented (e.g., intensive case management, therapeutic community, aftercare), as well as additional measurements and evaluation questions (note 3).

PAPERS IN THE PRESENT VOLUME

Table 1 summarizes the location of each study, the focus of the paper, client population, treatment groups, and follow-up rates. Although each

TABLE 1. Selected Characteristics of Studies

Authors/City	Study Focus	Sample	Groups	Follow up %
Sosin, Bruni, Ready Chicago	Program outcomes	n = 419 90% Black 75% male	1. intensive case management only 2. intensive case mgt with supported housing 3. usual care (control group)	74%
Lan, Jekel, Thompson, et al., New Haven	Program outcomes	n = 294 100% male 59% Black 19% Latino	1. day treatment in drug-free shelter 2. usual community services (control group)	80%
Lapham, Hall, Skipper Albuquerque	Program outcomes	n = 497 87% male 41% White 31% Hispanic 18% Nat. Am	1. high intensity–intensive case mgt/counseling+housing 2. medium intensity–peer support+housing 3. low intensity–motel-based housing (control group) 4. usual care–no housing (control group)	78%
North, Smith, Fox St. Louis	Program outcomes/ Dropout predictors	n = 149 100% women 97% Black 83% cocaine users	1. 90 day therapeutic community + aftercare 2. non-residential, day treatment (control group)	90%
Schumacher, Milby, Caldwell, et al. Birmingham	Dosage effects	n = 176 79% male 96% Black 72% cocaine users	1. enhanced care–day treatment⊳work therapy + housing 2. usual care–individual group counseling (control group)	74%
Braucht, Reichardt, Geissler, et al. Denver	Dosage effects/ Program outcomes	n = 323 85% male 56% White 29% Black 74% alcohol users	1. comprehensive residential/outpatient + intensive case mgt 2. usual care residential/outpatient (control group)	88%
Burnam, Morton, McGlynn, et al. Los Angeles	Program outcomes/ Dosage effects	n = 276 100% dually diagnosed 84% male 58% White 28% Black	1. social model residential treatment 2. non-residential social model 3. usual care (control group)	76%

Erickson, Stevens, McKnight, et al. Tucson	Motivation as outcome predictor	n = 494 89% male 40% White 60% alcohol users	1. 4 month modified therapeutic community 2. non-residential counseling/education (control group)	54%
Stahler, Shipley, Bartelt, DuCette Shandler Philadelphia	Client outcome predictors/ Program outcomes	n = 722 100% male 92% Black 77% cocaine users	1. residential treatment 2. shelter-based intensive case mgt 3. shelter-based usual care	76%
Wright, Devine New Orleans	Client outcome predictors/ Program outcomes	n = 670 75% male 82% Black 85% cocaine users	1. 12 month–extended care/independent living 2. 21 day transitional care 3. social detoxification (control group)	80%

project conducted a true experimental outcome evaluation of its intervention, there were considerable further analyses on important research questions. The papers that are included here represent important contributions to how best to serve homeless persons with substance abuse problems, and they address three vital areas in the field of substance abuse outcome research:

- evaluations of treatment effectiveness;
- dosage effects of services;
- client characteristic predictors of successful treatment.

The first four papers focus particularly on evaluation of program outcomes. Sosin, Bruni, and Reidy report on the effectiveness of a "progressive independence" model of treatment conducted in Chicago with homeless clients who are primarily male African-Americans.[15] This approach utilized outpatient treatment and 12-Step recovery groups with intensive case management focused on meeting the tangible needs of clients. Gradually, clients were expected to accept greater responsibility for their longer-term material needs. Experimental group subjects who received this treatment were found to have a greater reduction in substance use and better residential stability at the one year follow-up than clients in a control condition. This study underscores the necessity of combining treatment for substance abuse with an explicit focus on meeting the material needs of homeless clients.

Whereas the previous study recruited clients who had recently graduated from a short-term inpatient substance abuse program, Lam and her colleagues developed a program in New Haven that was provided in a shelter.[16] The Grant Street Partnership was a short-term shelter and day treatment program consisting of 90 days of residential treatment and six months of aftercare case management services serving primarily African-American and Latino homeless crack cocaine users. Compared to a usual services control group, the experimental group clients were more likely to maintain their abstinence over time and more likely to move into stable housing arrangements nine months after program entry. However, the control group did evidence considerable progress in terms of cocaine use reduction and residential stability.

This latter finding, that the control or comparison group clients improved from baseline to follow-up, appeared to be relatively common among the projects in this initiative (and will be discussed in more detail later). In Albuquerque, for example, Lapham, Hall, and Skipper report that their Project H&ART program, which compared four levels of intervention intensity involving case management, counseling, and housing, had similar findings.[17] With a population comprised mostly of a mix of homeless Caucasian, Hispanic, and Native American males with alcohol problems, the investigators found that all four groups (including the control group) improved significantly over time on a variety of outcome measures, but there were no differences in outcomes among the groups.

Similar findings are reported by Smith, North, and Fox with a population of homeless women with children in St. Louis.[18] Comparing a residential program using a modified therapeutic community approach versus non-residential services, clients in the former group were less likely to drop out but manifested no better outcomes than those in the non-residential group. However, as in the previously mentioned studies, clients in both groups improved significantly over time on drug use and housing stability.

Treatment effectiveness may not just be a function of the type of programmatic intervention, but a result of the amount of treatment exposure or dosage. Indeed, length of time spent in treatment, one measure of exposure, has been shown to be associated with outcome in a variety of treatment modalities.[19-22] Three papers in this issue address this question with different subject populations and treatment interventions.

Schumacher and his colleagues in Birmingham, with a homeless population composed primarily of male African-American cocaine users, found that more frequent attendance early in treatment resulted in better outcomes for a multifaceted day treatment program.[23] Braucht and his colleagues in Denver had similar findings with outpatient and residential treatment programs provided at Arapaho House.[24] With a study population comprised of mostly male, Caucasian alcoholics, they report that their clients improved significantly over time in terms of substance use, employment and housing status, physical and mental health, and quality of life. However, the effects were greatest at the end of the four month treatment period and diminished over time when the amount of services declined. This underscores the chronic nature of the problems that homeless substance abusers face, and the necessity for the continuity of treatment such as aftercare services to prevent relapse.

Finally, Burnam and her colleagues had similar results in Los Angeles with a largely white male, dually diagnosed subject population.[25] Clients were randomly assigned to three groups consisting of a social model residential program, a community-based nonresidential program, and a control group which accessed other community services. Similar to many of the other projects described, substance use and housing outcomes improved over time, but there were few differences among groups. As in the Denver project, length of time in residential treatment positively affected outcomes, but diminished over time.

Thus far, the major variables affecting outcomes have been type of programmatic intervention and program dose or exposure–both of which are treatment variables. However, there is a considerable literature concerning client variables that affect outcomes across a variety of treatment modalities.[26-28] Arguably one of the most important client variables is motivation for treatment. There has been substantial recent attention in the literature on the role of motivation in successful treatment.[29-34] In an attempt to ascertain the role of motivation in treatment outcomes, Erickson, Stevens, McKnight, and Figueredo used follow-up data on a sample of homeless predominantly male alcoholics (with a large proportion of Hispanics) who had been involved in a modified therapeutic community in Tucson. They found that greater motivation, readiness, and suitability for treatment, termed "willingness," was related to longer retention in the program and greater reduction of drug use.[35]

The final two papers focus on identifying client characteristics other than motivation that are associated with treatment outcome. Stahler, Shipley, Bartelt, and DuCette, working with a population of homeless primarily African-American crack addicted men in Philadelphia, identified several characteristics that were associated with successful outcomes.[36] Regardless of whether clients were treated in a residential facility or provided with case management services in a shelter, those who had lower recent and lifetime substance use, fewer prior treatment episodes for substance use, more stable housing, fewer incarcerations, and less social isolation tended to have more positive outcomes six months following treatment.

In the final paper in this volume, Wright and Devine examine predictors of outcomes for a sample of homeless mostly African-American crack cocaine users in New Orleans.[37] They found that stays in residential treatment of less than a few months provided virtually no improvement over detoxification only. The most robust predictor of treatment success was educational attainment, with those having a high school education or better manifesting better treatment outcomes. In addition, the investigators found similar results to the Philadelphia project concerning lower baseline substance use predicting lower follow-up use. That is, both studies appeared to confirm that past behavior is one of the best predictors of future behavior.

CONCLUSIONS

From the studies presented in this volume, there are a number of conclusions and issues that emerge:

1. It is essential to develop treatment programs that not only focus on the addiction but also address the tangible needs of homeless clients, particularly housing, income support, and employment.
2. Dropout rates are high for this population no matter what type of intervention was provided.[38] Part of the reason for this may be associated with a lack of motivation for treatment. Client motivation for program entry could have been associated with financial remuneration for research participation, obtaining shelter and food, taking a "break" from the streets or their addiction, etc. Since motivation for treatment seems to be positively related to retention and outcomes, there is therefore a need to develop flexible, low demand interventions which can accommodate clients who are not willing to initially commit to more extended care. Hopefully, clients can be gradually brought into more intensive treatment modalities when their motivation increases.
3. Clients in both experimental and control groups seemed to improve significantly by the end of treatment. However, with a few exceptions, treatment modality did not appear to differentially affect outcomes in most cases. There are several possible explanations. Since none of the control groups actually comprised a "no treatment" or placebo group, it could be that exposure to minimal services was as effective as exposure to a greater number of services. Many clients in the control conditions received 12-Step group interventions which may have had a particularly potent impact. In some of the studies,

control clients received a nearly equivalent quantity of services, only the type of treatment varied.

Another possible explanation concerns a regression to the mean effect in which clients tended to be recruited into treatment at their most acute phase of addiction, after they had "hit bottom" in many cases. Therefore it would be a natural progression for clients on average to improve over time. It may be that no matter what services are provided (or for that matter, no services), on average, clients will improve over time if they are assessed at baseline during an extreme point in their addiction and life functioning. Clearly, these possible explanations require further investigation.

4. Treatment outcomes appeared to be particularly positive after treatment, but seemed to diminish over time. This suggests the need for longer-term, continuous interventions for this population. Aftercare needs to address not only the maintenance of sobriety, but also the tangible needs and social isolation of clients. For example, self-help groups could be used to augment other aftercare interventions to reduce the pervasive social isolation many clients experience after leaving treatment.

5. It appears that there are certain subgroups of clients who will have more positive outcomes than others, most notably those with higher educational attainment, with less severe substance use, less criminal involvement, and those who are less socially isolated. This type of information may be useful for matching clients to appropriate treatment services.

In conclusion, homeless individuals who enter treatment programs for their substance abuse problems also come with a multiplicity of other problems which further complicates their clinical picture: they are invariably poor, often in poor health, residentially unstable, usually unemployed, frequently victims as well as perpetrators of criminal activity, usually cross-addicted to other substances, socially isolated, and frequently suffer from psychiatric comorbidities. Because of these concomitant problems and characteristics, they represent one of the greatest challenges to substance abuse treatment providers.

Thus far, there has been a paucity of empirical research on how to best provide treatment for this indigent population. Hopefully, this volume will help to begin to fill this gap and contribute to our ability to develop and evaluate more responsive treatment models for serving homeless individuals with substance abuse problems. The papers in this volume have begun to identify types of program interventions, client characteristics, and dosage of treatment as correlates of outcome. Future research should not only focus on these discrete factors, but must look at the interactions among them. We cannot assume that "one size fits all" in addictions treatment. We must begin to identify which types of clients seem to do well with which types of programs with what amounts of exposure. Only once we have broadened our knowledge base to account for this level of complexity in service programming can we truly tailor our treatment programs to best meet the needs of our clients.

Gerald J. Stahler, PhD
Department of Geography and Urban Studies
Temple University

NOTES

1. One of the fourteen projects was terminated after the first year. The three other projects not included in this volume could not meet the publication time constraints since they were either undertaking further analyses or data collection.

2. At least three other volumes have been published concerning various aspects of treating *homeless* substance abusers stemming from the two NIAAA/NIDA initiatives. *Alcoholism Treatment Quarterly* published an issue describing nine demonstration projects funded by NIAAA in an earlier initiative but they did not report outcome results.[39] A second volume of *Alcoholism Treatment Quarterly* described the implementation after the first year of funding of the substance abuse treatment programs presented in this issue.[40] Finally, a special issue of *Contemporary Drug Problems* reports qualitative findings from some of the projects described in this volume.[41] However, the present book is thus far the only one to focus on the quantitative outcome results of programs designed to serve homeless substance abusers.

3. As this volume goes to press, Robert Orwin and his associates at R.O.W. Sciences in collaboration with David Cordray and his colleagues at Vanderbilt's Institute for Public Policy Studies, are utilizing sophisticated meta-analytic statistical techniques on individual level data to synthesize the results across all of the sites. The results should be completed by the beginning of 1996.

REFERENCES

1. Fischer P. Estimating prevalence of alcohol, drug, and mental health problems in the contemporary homeless population: A review of the literature. Contemp Drug Probl 1989; 16:333-390.

2. Fischer P, Breakey W. The epidemiology of alcohol, drug, and mental disorders among homeless persons. Am Psychol 1991; 46:1115-1128.

3. Lehman AF, Cordray DS. Prevalence of alcohol, drug, and mental disorders among the homeless: One more time. Contemp Drug Probl 1993; 20: 355-384.

4. Jenks C. The homeless. Cambridge, MA: Harvard University Press, 1994.

5. Milburn NJ, Booth JA. Illicit drug and alcohol use among homeless black adults in shelters. Drugs Soc 1992; 6:115-155.

6. Spinner GF, Leaf PJ. Homelessness and drug abuse in New Haven. Hosp Community Psychiatry 1992; 43:166-168.

7. Stahler GJ, Cohen E. Homelessness and substance abuse in the 1980s. Contemp Drug Probl 1995; 22:in press.

8. Susser E, Struening EL, Conover S. Psychiatric problems in homeless men. Arch Gen Psychiatry 1989; 46:845-850.

9. Institute of Medicine. Homelessness, health, and human needs. Washington, D.C.: National Academy Press, 1988.

10. Robertson MJ, Zlotnick C, Westerfelt A. Homeless adults: A special population in public alcohol treatment programs. Contemp Drug Probl 1993; 20: 499-520.

11. Breakey W. Treating the homeless. Alcohol Health Res World 1987; 11: 42-47.

12. McLellan AT, Luborsky L, O'Brien CP, Woody G. An improved evaluation instrument for substance abuse patients: The addiction severity index. J Nerv Ment Dis 1980; 168:26-33.

13. Skinner HA, Horn JL. Alcohol dependence scale user's guide. Toronto: Addiction Research Foundation.

14. Barrow SM, Hellman F, Lovell AM, et al. Personal history form. Community Support Systems Evaluation Program, Epidemiology of Mental Disorders Research Department. New York: New York State Psychiatric Institute, 1985.

15. Sosin MR, Bruni M, Reidy M. Paths and impacts in the Progressive Independence Model: A homelessness and substance abuse intervention in Chicago. J Addict Dis 1995; 14:1-20.

16. Lam JA, Jekel JF, Thompson, KS, et al. Assessing the value of a short-term residential drug treatment program for homeless men. J Addict Dis 1995; 14:21-39.

17. Lapham SC, Hall M, Skipper BJ. Homelessness and substance use among alcohol abusers following participation in Project H&ART. J Addict Dis 1995; 14:41-55.

18. Smith EM, North CS, Fox LW. Eighteen-month follow-up data on a treatment program for homeless substance abusing mothers. J Addict Dis 1995; 14:57-72.

19. Allison M, Hubbard RL. Drug abuse treatment process: A review of the literature. Int J Addict 1985; 20:1321-1345.

20. Condelli WS, Hubbard, RL. Relationship between time spent in treatment and client outcomes from therapeutic communities. J Subst Abuse Treat 1994; 11:25-33.

21. Simpson DD. The relation of time spent in drug abuse treatment to post-treatment outcome. Am J Psychiatry 1979; 136:1449-1453.

22. Simpson DD. Treatment for drug abuse: Follow-up outcomes and length of time spent. Arch Gen Psychiatry 1981; 38:875-880.

23. Schumacher JE, Milby JB, Caldwell E, et al. Treatment outcome as a function of treatment attendance with homeless persons abusing cocaine. J Addict Dis 1995: 14:73-85.

24. Braucht GN, Reichardt CS, Geissler LJ, et al. Effective services for homeless substance abusers. J Addict Dis 1995; 14:87-109.

25. Burnam MA, Morton SC, McGlynn EA, et al. An experimental evaluation of residential and nonresidential treatment for dually diagnosed homeless adults. J Addict Dis 1995; 14:111-134.

26. McLellan AT. Patient characteristics associated with outcome. In Cooper JR, Altman F, Brown BS, Czechowicz D, eds. Research on the treatment of narcotic addiction: State of the art. Rockville, MD: National Institute on Drug Abuse, 1991:500-529.

27. Means L, Small M, Dapone D, et al. Client demographics and outcome in outpatient cocaine treatment. Int J Addict 1989; 24:765-783.

28. Stark, MJ. Dropping out of substance abuse treatment: A clinically-oriented review. Clin Psychol Rev 1992; 12:93-116.

29. Snow MG, Prochaska JO, Rossi JS. Processes of change in Alcoholics Anonymous: Maintenance factors in long-term sobriety. J Stud Alcohol 1994; 55:362-371.

30. DeLeon G, Jainchill N. Circumstances, motivation, readiness, and suitability as correlates of tenure in treatment. J Psychoactive Drugs 1986; 18:203-208.

31. Miller W. Motivation for treatment: A review with special emphasis on alcoholism. Psychol Bull 1985; 98:84-107.

32. Prochaska JO, DiClemente CC, Norcross JC. In search of how people change: Applications to addictive behaviors. Am Psychol 1992; 47:1102-1114.

33. Simpson DD, Joe GW. Motivation as a predictor of early dropout from drug abuse treatment. Psychother 1993; 30:357-368.

34. Stahler, G, Cohen, E, Greene, M, et al. A qualitative study of treatment success among homeless crack addicted men: Definitions and attributions. Contemp Drug Probl 1995; 22:in press.

35. Erickson JR, Stevens S, McKnight P, Figueredo AJ. Willingness for treatment as a predictor of retention and outcomes. J Addict Dis 1995; 14:135-150.

36. Stahler GJ, Shipley, Jr., TE, Bartelt D, DuCette JP, Shandler, IW. Evaluating alternative treatments for homeless substance-abusing men: Outcomes and predictors of success. J Addict Dis 1995; 14:151-167.

37. Wright JD, DeVine JA. Factors that interact with treatment to predict outcomes in substance abuse programs for the homeless. J Addict Dis 1995; 14:169-181.

38. Stahler GJ, Shipley TE, Bartelt D, et al. Retention issues in treating homeless polydrug users: Philadelphia. Alcohol Treat Q 1993; 10:201-216.

39. Argeriou M, McCarty D, eds. Treating alcoholism and drug abuse among homeless men and women: Nine community demonstration grants [special issue]. Alcohol Treat Q 1990; 7(1).

40. Conrad K, Hultman C, Lyons J, eds. Treatment of the chemically dependent homeless: Theory and implementation in fourteen American projects. New York: Haworth Press, 1993.

41. Stahler GJ, Cohen E, eds. Homelessness and substance abuse in the 1990s: Qualitative studies from service demonstration projects. Cont Drug Probl [special issue] 1995; 22(2).

Paths and Impacts
in the Progressive Independence Model:
A Homelessness
and Substance Abuse Intervention
in Chicago

Michael R. Sosin, PhD
Maria Bruni, AM
Mairead Reidy, PhD

SUMMARY. In an attempt to reduce homelessness and substance abuse, Chicago graduates of short-term inpatient substance abuse programs who lacked domiciles were placed into one of three conditions: (1) a case management only intervention (n = 96), (2) a case management with supported housing intervention (n = 136), or (3) a control condition (n = 187) that allowed access to normal aftercare in the community. The two treatment interventions used a "progressive independence" approach, which focuses on simultaneously amelio-

The authors are affiliated with The University of Chicago. Michael R. Sosin is Professor, Maria Bruni is Research Assistant, and Mairead Reidy is Research Coordinator.

Address corrspondence to Michael Sosin, PhD, Professor, School of Social Service Administration, University of Chicago, 969 East 60th Street, Chicago, Illinois 60637.

This paper was prepared in part under grant number AA08773 from the National Institute of Alcohol Abuse and Alcoholism. The conclusions are those of the authors.

[Haworth co-indexing entry note]: "Paths and Impacts in the Progressive Independence Model: A Homelessness and Substance Abuse Intervention in Chicago." Sosin, Michael R., Maria Bruni, and Mairead Reidy. Co-published simultaneously in the *Journal of Addictive Diseases* (The Haworth Medical Press, an imprint of The Haworth Press, Inc.) Vol. 14, No. 4, 1995, pp. 1-20; and: *The Effectiveness of Social Interventions for Homeless Substance Abusers* (ed: Gerald J. Stahler) The Haworth Medical Press, an imprint of The Haworth Press, Inc., 1995, pp. 1-20. Single or multiple copies of this article are available from The Haworth Document Delivery Service [1-800-342-9678; 9:00 a.m. - 5:00 p.m. (EST)].

1

rating tangible needs and clinical problems. Multivariate analyses suggest that subjects in both treatment interventions experienced lower levels of substance abuse and higher levels of residential stability than subjects in the control condition, as measured over the course of a year. Further analysis suggests that retention was improved by the focus on immediate tangible resources, substance abuse was reduced by both the support of outpatient substance abuse treatment and the promulgation of changes in coping styles, and residential stability was increased by both the focus on access to income maintenance benefits and help with location of housing. *[Article copies available from The Haworth Document Delivery Service: 1-800-342-9678.]*

Adults who are homeless are thought to be particularly unlikely to benefit from substance abuse treatment. Allegedly, their immediate tangible concerns and longer-term housing problems are sufficiently overwhelming to limit their acceptance of treatment, as well as their commitment to recovery if they do enroll. Their progress is said to be further reduced by the many barriers to the success of any possible interventions aimed at the complicating residential problem: members of the population may suffer from deficient social support systems, the tendency to withdraw from supports, the lack of stable sources of income, limited access to low-cost housing, or certain psychological problems.[1-6] Indeed, some program directors say that amelioration of homelessness demands such a focus on tangible supports and related services that it compromises the full dedication to recovery from substance abuse.[7-10]

The "progressive independence" model developed by The University of Chicago and Travelers and Immigrants Aid of Chicago[11,12] is based on the premise that it is possible to provide immediate tangible resources while also supporting further treatment for abuse and other relevant personal and situational problems. The model calls for the immediate provision of any needed transportation tokens, food vouchers, medical care, and furniture and rent deposits (for those with long-term ability to support themselves). However, under the assumption that clients should be more fully able to commit to recovery when materially stable, provision is conditioned on attendance in outpatient and Alcoholics Anonymous meetings in the community. Individuals are also required to progressively take responsibility for other activities needed to address their problems, such as obtaining employment, work training, or if neither is available, welfare benefits (obtained with the help of intensive advocacy made available by the project); attending the project's group and individual counseling concerning intrapersonal, relationship, and permanent housing issues; and cooperating with a cognitive behavioral relapse prevention model that is utilized by the case managers. The clients also must remain abstinent from drugs and alcohol, and must sign a contract agreeing to cooperate with the (negotiated) treatment plan. Those who do not keep these agreements are first confronted with their behavior; if the problems continue, the clients are suspended and eventually asked to withdraw. In sum, the model is consistent with the above-mentioned literature on causes of homelessness; with suggestions that economic, residential, and family stability aid recovery from substance abuse;[13-15] with basic principles of substance abuse interventions; and with our claim that help with tangible needs can and should be balanced with expectations for substance abuse treatment.[12]

In an experiment based on this model, clients finishing a short-term (21- to 28-day) treatment program were assigned to either one of two experimental interventions or to a control condition. The *case management only* intervention provided the progressive independence case management services under a scheme in which workers also helped clients find housing in the community. The *housing* intervention provided the case management model along with supported housing in one of three blocks of twenty apartments, found in recently renovated buildings serving those with low incomes. Both interventions were meant to last for up to eight months, although less intensive case management services could (but rarely did) last longer. Those who suffered two relapses or repeatedly violated program rules could not remain in the housing. They could continue case management as long as they agreed to a new contract that would guard against further relapses. The clients placed in the *control* condition were referred by the relevant short-term program staff to an outpatient or inpatient substance abuse agency, to welfare offices (as needed), and to an address of some kind. In the current paper, we ask whether, and by what mechanisms, each of the two treatment interventions reduced substance abuse and homelessness beyond the progress achieved by individuals placed in the control condition.

DATA AND METHODS

Subjects

The recruitment sites included two of Chicago men's and one women's short-term substance abuse programs in which indigent clients enroll after completing week-long detoxification treatment. Recruitment occurred between May, 1991, and October, 1992. Program graduates were deemed eligible if they met any one of the following criteria: (1) having a recent history of substantial homelessness (four months in the last two years, including time living with relatives but moving at least every thirty days), (2) being homeless at the time of entry into treatment, or (3) being in imminent danger of homelessness upon program completion (this was a rarely met criterion). Thirty four percent of short-term program graduates were found eligible.

Potential subjects who agreed to participate were enrolled in one of the three conditions. Assignment rotated so that those entering the short-term programs in a particular two-week period were eligible for a single condition. Rotation was regular in the first few months and random afterwards, guaranteeing that assignment approached a randomized design. This technique was used to assuage concerns that disruptions of the short-term programs would occur if members of a single cohort received different treatment options.

By design, the number of rounds of recruitment varied for each condition. This was meant to compensate for possible differences in acceptance and follow-up rates: those in the case management condition might reject the services immediately, while those in the control group might be more difficult to attract for later follow-up interviews. Because subjects in the case management only condition rejected services at an even greater than expected rate, recruitment for this intervention was continued for two extra months at two of the three sites. To compensate for the resulting difference in probabilities of entering a given condition by short-term site, responses of clients within a condition were weighted in inverse proportion to the number of two-week periods for which their short-term program was eligible. Forty-nine individuals refused the original screening for homelessness or assignment into groups. Of the remainder, 96 accepted at least some case management only services, 136 accepted some services in the housing condition, and 187 individuals entered the control condition. These represent 34%, 91%, and 100% of those offered enrollment in each of the three conditions.

The average length of care was three months in the case management only condition and six months in the housing condition. While the experiment was not premised on the assumption that completion of the full eight months of services was expected, 78% of case management only clients and 58% of housing clients left prior to this point. Acceptance and retention seem to be at or above the mean for substance abuse programs despite the apparently low rates.[16] This may be attributed either to a greater motivation for treatment than predicted by the literature on homelessness,[17,18] or to the model's emphasis on recruiting aggressively and providing tangible and recreational services. Analyses suggest that these services indeed improved retention.[12]

Data

A baseline interview was conducted near the time clients were completing the short-term program. A first follow-up interview was scheduled six months later; a second follow-up interview was scheduled six months after that. Individuals who agreed to follow-up interviews were pursued with vigor. They were given appointments; were sent reminder postcards and bus tokens; knew they would be paid $15 and $20 for the interviews (they were paid $10 for the first); were asked to call in periodically to report their address; were given an additional $1 for each requested call; knew that one randomly selected subject who called in each three-month period was given an extra $20; and were tracked through contacts they provided, voting records, and other lists. Two staff members routinely searched shelters and meal programs. Biweekly visits were made to the county jail during the last year. The overall response rate was 77.8% for the first follow-up interview and 73.7% for the second.

CLIENT AND PROGRAM CHARACTERISTICS

Overall Characteristics

Characteristics of the obtained population are summarized in Table 1, which like the ensuing tables includes those individuals who accepted their assigned condition. As noted, the average age of the subjects is about 35, the educational level averages slightly less than twelve years, while 26 percent are female. Fifty percent say they were homeless only once. Reported homelessness over the course of adult life averages 26 months. These characteristics match those of an earlier sample of Chicago homeless adults who used shelters or meal programs.[19] While a somewhat high 90 percent of the current population is African-American (compared to 74 percent in the previous study), this reflects the locales of the programs from which recruitment occurred.

Typical members of the current sample report three treatment episodes for alcohol abuse and two for drug abuse. This includes the stays in the short-term programs from which they were recruited. Roughly seventy-five percent of sample members report suffering from alcohol abuse. Confirming service provider beliefs that polydrug abuse is a common pattern among those who are homeless in Chicago, a similar proportion reports drug abuse. Cocaine was the most commonly mentioned drug.

TABLE 1. Description of Sample (N).

	Total	Housing	Case Management	Control
Average Age	35.0 (417)	35.5 (135)	35.2 (96)	34.6 (187)
Education	11.8 (418)	11.7 (135)	11.9 (96)	11.8 (187)
Percent Female	25.5 (419)	28.5 (136)	24.2 (96)	24.1 (187)
Percent Black	89.9 (418)	89.8 (136)	90.4 (95)	89.8 (187)
Percent With Only One Homeless Spell	50.2 (384)	46.5 (125)	51.4 (91)	52.2 (168)
Average Months of Homeless Experience	25.7 (419)	27.1 (136)	25.2 (96)	24.9 (187)
Lived with Other Adults Prior to Most Recent Homeless Spell	76.5 (382)	77.8 (124)	73.7 (90)	77.1 (168)
Average Number of Alcohol Treatments	2.7 (407)	3.5 (129)	2.7 (95)	2.3 (183)
Average Number of Drug Treatments	2.3 (411)	2.2 (131)	2.9 (95)	2.1 (185)
Average Days Using Alcohol/Drugs in Past 30 at Baseline	17.5 (404)	17.8 (131)	16.9 (91)	16.4 (182)
Days Domiciled in Past 60 at Baseline	18.0 (386)	14.9 (127)	20.5 (85)	18.9 (174)
Average Days Using Alcohol/Drugs in Past 30 at Second Follow-Up**	5.5 (304)	4.8 (111)	4.3 (72)	6.8 (121)
Days Domiciled in Past 60 at Second Follow-Up**	39.0 (299)	40.5 (108)	41.7 (70)	36.0 (121)

For Comparison Among Groups: *p < .05; **p < .01

The vast majority of members of the current sample (76.5%) say they lived with other adults before their last spell of homelessness. Slightly over half of the time reported homeless (28 days) in the last two months was spent moving from relative to relative. This degree of contact with others surpasses that of the sample of shelter and meal program users. Reported incomes are also higher on average. However, such characteristics seem common in samples of users of alcohol and drug treatment programs; service users may enter care due to the demands of the relatives to whom they are attached, as well as due to their special skills in obtaining resources.[20,21]

Group Differences

As Table 1 also reports, chi-square and analysis of variance tests find that individuals who enroll in each of the three treatment conditions have similar demographic traits, substance abuse histories, homelessness histories, and family composition. There thus are few obvious differences on conventionally measured variables. Nevertheless, below we search to find and control for further differences, reducing possible biases that can affect the measurement of treatment effects.

Criterion Variables

Criterion variables represent scores on substance abuse and housing stability. These are calculated not just for program graduates, but for all individuals who agreed to begin their assigned intervention. Inclusion occurs because all had an opportunity to be affected by treatment. Indeed, because early exits could reflect programmatic decisions to expel those who continue to consume alcohol or drugs, exclusion of early leavers would distort the analysis of outcomes.

The outcome analyses make use of variables gathered from the second follow-up interviews, which occurred six to nine months after the treatment interventions typically ceased (one year after recruitment). Substance abuse is measured by an average of reported days using alcohol, and days using drugs, in the thirty days prior to this interview. The use of an average limits the number of outcome variables considered in this article. Housing stability is measured as the number of days subjects report being in a stable domicile in the sixty prior to the interview. Stability, in turn, is defined as the number of days on which individuals paid rent or resided with friends or relatives on a permanent basis. Reported days of literal homelessness is not used because it has a more skewed distribution. When using alternate measures, analyses suggest that alcohol abuse is affected by the interventions somewhat more than is drug abuse, especially by the housing program. Preliminary statistical analyses suggest that the measure of homelessness and residential stability bear similar relations to the interventions.

In any case, there is vast improvement on each criterion variable between the baseline and second follow-up interview. As Table 1 suggests, reported days using substances decreases from an average of 17.5 to 5.5; reported days domiciled increases from 18.0 to 39.0. However, large and statistically significant changes even occur among the members of the control group. This may be attributed to the motivation reflected in the decision to use short-term treatment programs; to the impact of these short-term programs; and to regression towards the mean. Such changes in the control group set an upper bound to any possible treatment effects.

OUTCOME ANALYSIS

The analyses of outcomes are presented in Tables 2 and 3. Each column of each of the tables reports ordinary least squares regressions in which binary variables represent the case management only and supported housing interventions. The binary variable representing membership in the control condition is excluded. As a result, the unstandardized regression coefficients attached to the indicators of the interventions indicate the impact of each intervention compared to progress of members of the control group; the coefficients indicate reported days of alcohol or drug consumption, and reported days of residential stability, that can be accounted for by each of the interventions. We rely on one-tailed significance tests (and the .05 level of statistical significance) when testing the prior hypotheses that the interventions are efficacious. Two-tailed tests are used elsewhere.

Control Variables

In the analyses reported in column 1 of each table, one control variable involves the length of time from the baseline to the second follow-up interview, which can vary due to difficulties in finding individuals and scheduling interviews. A second includes the number of days in the relevant period spent in such a controlled environment as a prison or mental hospital. While the average is small (2.4 out of the last 30 days; 6.7 out of the last 60), inclusion of the latter controls for the number of days in settings in which individuals cannot drink or use drugs and are neither truly domiciled nor homeless.

Analyses in column 1 also control for characteristics found to vary across the three treatment conditions. These were determined by a procedure that (1) searched for statistically significant group differences (chi-square or F-tests) among 94 variables representing individual demographic traits, personal deficits, proclivities, and resources; (2) conducted a multinominal regression of the variables with statistically significant zero order relations; and (3) excluded variables that had no predictive power in distinguishing either treatment group from the control group, or in contributing to the model as a whole, at the .10 level or below. Six baseline interview variables were identified and serve as controls. These include: being recruited from one particular short-term program, reported perception of health problems at the baseline on a five point scale,[22] whether the individual had access to an automobile, having ever been married, having foster care experience as a child, and having lived with one's mother continuously up until age eighteen. The variables reduce the -2 log-likelihood in the multinominal analysis from 886 to 826.

Other control variables stemming from the baseline interview, which are summarized in the tables, represent factors which the literature suggests predict the criterion variables. Inclusion increases the precision of the estimation and also helps contribute to knowledge about reasons for continued substance abuse and homelessness. Further precision is achieved by controlling for the baseline level of days of substance abuse or days in housing, and the interaction of each of the two treatment conditions by the relevant baseline trait. The latter variables are centered to reduce multicollinearity.[23]

Sample Selection

Column 2 of each table adds to the above variables a control for bias resulting from non-response to the follow-up interview. This control variable, called lambda, represents a so-called Heckman correction.[24] This (under certain statistical assumptions) allows for unbiased estimates of the remaining regression coefficients. The term represents the density of failing to respond to the second interview, divided by one minus the distribution of this variable. The density and distribution come from a probit equation modeling non-response with (in our case) the control variables listed above, the variables representing the housing and case management only conditions (those once in the interventions should be easier to find), age, sex, race, previous alcohol and drug use, previous months of homelessness, season of the first interview (individuals baselined in different seasons are contacted in different months for follow-up interviews and respond differentially, perhaps due to the weather), the identity of the baseline interviewer (personal style of a few interviewers increased follow-up), a measure of anxiety stemming from a factor analysis of the General Health Questionnaire (GHQ),[25,12] perceived physical health problems on a five point scale (individuals with problems are less likely to respond to the follow-up interview), previous military experience, previous receipt of welfare benefits, months in the longest job, the number of friends and family members who usually know the subject's whereabouts (each measures attachment to other

TABLE 2. Alcohol and Drug Use at Second Follow-Up Interview: OLS Models Uncorrected and Corrected for Sample Selection (t value).

	1. N = 294	2. N = 286	3. N = 253	4. N = 245
INTERVENTION				
Housing Condition	-1.999†	-2.316*	-0.815	-1.031
	(-1.89)	(-2.07)	(-.67)	(-.85)
Case Managment Only Condition	-2.461*	-2.534*	-0.481	-0.416
	(-2.01)	(-2.08)	(-.35)	(-.31)
Constant	8.048	7.840	10.087	10.570*
	(1.87)	(1.82)	(1.85)	(1.99)
CONTROL VARIABLES				
Time Between Baseline and Second Follow-Up	0.010*	0.010*	0.007	0.006
	(2.40)	(2.38)	(1.46)	(1.45)
Days in a Controlled Environment in Past 30	-0.166*	-0.151*	-0.171*	-0.152
	(-2.30)	(-2.07)	(-2.13)	(-1.89)
Recruitment from Veterans' Alcohol Program	0.427	0.622	1.361	1.642
	(.35)	(.51)	(.97)	(1.19)
Health Problems at Baseline	-0.061	-0.159	-0.101	-0.185
	(-.06)	(-.16)	(-.09)	(-.17)
Have Access to Car	-2.151	-2.221	-2.439	-2.637
	(-1.67)	(-1.74)	(-1.68)	(-1.88)
Ever Married	-0.919	-0.893	-1.171	-1.326
	(-.96)	(-.93)	(-1.13)	(-1.31)
Foster Care as Child	1.744	1.986	2.158	2.373
	(1.24)	(1.43)	(1.37)	(1.57)
Lived with Mother until age 18	0.321	0.469	-0.280	-0.109
	(.33)	(.47)	(-.26)	(-.10)
Female	1.359	1.251	1.142	0.835
	(1.23)	(1.14)	(.94)	(.70)

GHQ Self-Esteem Scale	-0.305** (-3.24)	-0.295** (-3.18)	-0.248* (-2.28)	-0.244* (-2.33)
GHQ Depression Scale	-0.657* (-2.03)	-0.687* (-2.14)	-0.815* (-2.31)	-0.856* (-2.49)
GHQ Anxiety Scale	0.221* (2.25)	0.227* (2.32)	0.260* (2.42)	0.272 (2.57)
ASI Legal Problems Composite Score	8.028** (2.96)	8.500** (3.17)	5.462 (1.88)	5.806* (2.06)
Days Using Alcohol/Drugs in Past 30 at Baseline	0.099 (1.22)	0.090 (1.13)	0.036 (.41)	0.035 (.41)
Housing—Alcohol/Drug Use at Baseline Interaction	0.087 (.76)	0.096 (.84)	0.117 (.95)	0.130 (1.09)
CMO—Alcohol/Drug Use at Baseline Interaction	-0.109 (-.87)	-0.090 (-.73)	-0.028 (-.21)	-0.005 (-0.035)
Lambda	--	0.182 (.10)	--	-0.378 (-.20)
MEDIATING FACTORS				
Outpatient Services at First Follow-Up	--	--	-0.746** (-2.68)	-0.785** (-2.92)
Avoidance Coping at First Follow-Up	--	--	0.206* (2.02)	0.225* (2.26)
Active Coping at First Follow-Up	--	--	-0.151 (-1.13)	-0.148 (-1.12)

Notes:
For two-tailed significance test: *p < .05; **p < .01; ***p < .001
For one-tailed significance test of treatment conditions: †p < .05

TABLE 3. Days Domiciled in Past 60 at Second Follow-up Interview: OLS Model Uncorrected and Corrected for Sample Selection (t value).

	1. N = 259	2. N = 251	3. N = 249	4. N = 241
INTERVENTION				
Housing Condition	6.422*	5.822†	4.229	3.986
	(2.00)	(1.73)	(1.24)	(1.14)
Case Management Only Condition	8.650*	8.474*	6.365	6.419†
	(2.35)	(2.30)	(1.62)	(1.65)
Constant	39.316***	40.828***	38.627***	39.286***
	(5.50)	(5.35)	(4.98)	(4.76)
CONTROL VARIABLES				
Time Between Baseline and Second Follow-Up Interview	-0.012	-0.011	-0.018	-0.018
	(-.97)	(-.93)	(-1.39)	(-1.37)
Days in a Controlled Environment in Past 60	-0.817***	-0.816***	-0.810***	-0.808***
	(-9.53)	(-9.38)	(-8.95)	(-8.82)
Recruitment from Veteran's Alcohol Program	4.686	4.768	2.438	2.199
	(1.33)	(1.33)	(.66)	(.578)
Health Problems at Baseline	1.082	0.879	0.648	0.469
	(.36)	(.29)	(.21)	(.154)
Have Access to Car	2.323	1.970	1.604	1.447
	(.60)	(.52)	(.40)	(.37)
Ever Married	-0.062	-0.545	-0.122	-0.444
	(-.02)	(-.19)	(-.04)	(-.15)
Foster Care as Child	-5.869	-6.019	-4.542	-4.607
	(-1.41)	(-1.44)	(-1.05)	(-1.08)
Lived with Mother until age 18	-1.257	-1.807	-0.887	-1.319
	(-.43)	(-.610)	(-.29)	(-.44)
Female	3.162	2.756	2.038	1.566
	(.88)	(.772)	(.54)	(.42)

12

Number of Homeless Spells in Past Five Years	1.411	1.431	1.849	1.890
	(1.85)	(1.92)	(1.67)	(1.76)
Income Maintenance Benefits at Baseline ($)	1.105	1.097	0.788	0.834
	(1.45)	(1.42)	(.99)	(1.06)
Days Using Alcohol/Drugs in Past 30 at Baseline	0.146	0.151*	0.151	0.152*
	(1.89)	(1.97)	(1.91)	(1.96)
Days Domiciled in Past 60 at Baseline	0.135	0.146	0.136	0.145
	(1.42)	(1.58)	(1.40)	(1.53)
Housing–Days Domiciled in Past 60 at Baseline Interaction	-0.183	-0.186	-0.179	-0.176
	(-1.25)	(-1.28)	(-1.18)	(-1.18)
CMO–Days Domiciled in Past 60 at Baseline Interaction	-0.277	-0.292	-0.242	-0.258
	(-1.76)	(-1.89)	(-1.51)	(-1.64)
Lambda	--	-3.170	--	-1.305
		(-.60)		(-.24)
MEDIATING FACTORS				
Employment Services at First Follow-Up	--	--	1.032	0.909
			(.54)	(.48)
Income Maintenance Benefits ($) at First Follow-Up	--	--	0.927*	0.914*
			(2.01)	(1.99)

Notes:
For two-tailed significance test: *p < .05; **p < .01; ***p < .001
For one-tailed significance test of treatment conditions: †p < .05

people and relates to improved follow up), and perceived desirability of counseling for employment problems on a five point scale (which perhaps leads to a greater interest in talking to the interviewer). The probit model reduces the -2 log-likelihood from 441 to 349.

Columns 3 and 4 repeat the analyses described above while adding variables representing possible mediating factors. These are first follow-up scores on certain factors that represent the many changes expected to be brought about by the interventions. In particular, substance abuse should be reduced by the use of outpatient services, as well as by the changes in personal coping style brought about by required counseling; homelessness should be reduced by improved access to work and welfare benefits. Use of first follow-up scores on the relevant variables is appropriate because most or all of the intensive intervention was completed by this time.

Substance Use Findings

General Findings. Results reported in column 1 of Table 2 suggest that the case management only intervention decreases reported average days of alcohol and drug consumption by a modest, but statistically significant 2.5 days; the housing intervention decreases the variable by a statistically significant 2 days. Other statistically significant coefficients suggest that substance consumption is greater when there is more time between interviews, as well as when there are fewer days in which the subject lived in a controlled environment.

As might be expected, statistically significant coefficients also suggest that substance consumption is lower for subjects who have higher levels of self-esteem and lower levels of anxiety as measured on the baseline interview. But results also suggest that consumption is lower for those with high depression scores at the baseline. The latter relation, which is loosely anticipated by other literature,[26] may indicate that depression leads to a greater awareness of the effects of drinking or drug use on moods, and thus to a more complete commitment to abstinence. A final statistically significant relation suggests that consumption is higher for those with greater involvement with the legal system (as measured by the ASI legal composite score).[21] Legal problems may lead to stress that limits recovery, or may indicate commitment to a lifestyle that also includes use of alcohol and drugs. Column 2 suggests that sample selection bias is not sufficient to alter the statistical significance of any coefficient.

Mediation. Previously constructed analyses[10] of first follow-up interviews suggest that the interventions affect a number of relevant, potentially mediating factors. Both interventions improve reported active behavioral coping scores beyond levels of the control group (as measured by scores developed from a factor analysis).[10,13] These changes suggest improvements in the tendency to talk to someone about problems or crises. The case management only intervention also reduces first follow-up interview scores of reliance on avoidance coping, suggesting a reduction in the tendency to deny problems. Previous analyses also suggest that each intervention improves the number of types of outpatient alcohol and drug services used at the first follow-up interview. All such relations confirm that the major components of the intervention are operating; the counseling techniques are aimed at improving such coping responses to triggers for use of alcohol and drugs, while use of other services was encouraged (it was mandated) by the interventions. These components are expected to affect substance abuse on the basis of previous literature suggesting the role of coping styles and continuance in treatment.[13,16,27,28]

The results of an equation adding the mediating factors are listed in column 3 of Table 2. The table indeed suggests that days of consumption at the second follow-up interview are reduced for subjects whose avoidance coping scores were lower at the first follow-up interview, as well as for those who used more outpatient services at the first follow-up interview. Addition of the coping and service use variables to the equation predicting second follow-up substance consumption also reduces the effects of both interventions to a point at which their coefficients fail to reach statistical significance. While not presented in the table, further analysis suggests that the addition of the measure of alcohol and drug use at the first follow-up also eliminates the statistical significance of the coefficients attached to the interventions. It even eliminates the significance of the coefficients attached to avoidance coping and outpatient services. It thus may be that the mediating variables reduce alcohol and drug use by the time treatment was completed, and that the reduction is sustained to the time of the final interview.

Column 4 of Table 2 again suggests that sample bias has a small impact on any of the main findings. At most, there are changes in statistical significance for two variables whose levels of statistical significance fluctuate quite near the .05 level.

Residential Stability Results

Basic Results. Table 3 reports the regression equations predicting the number of days in which respondents report being stably domiciled in the sixty before the second follow-up interview. As noted in the first column, the case management intervention increases residential stability by a statistically significant 9 days (rounded); the housing intervention also shows effectiveness, albeit to a slightly lesser degree (6 days). The difference between the two interventions is indeed surprising. Perhaps, as the treatment staff believe, housing residents are more difficult to motivate to search for future residences when they are in supported dwellings (just as they seem to less fully eliminate avoidance coping strategies as measured at the first follow-up interview). They may also be less adept at remaining in the community upon release, in that they do not receive most of their services in this location. For example, the tangible aid they receive when in the housing program may not help them find community housing; their somewhat lower propensity to receive income maintenance benefits (as discussed below) may limit the cash available for housing.

The only control variable that predicts second follow-up interview residential stability (to a statistically significant degree) is residence in a controlled environment. Such weak effects might occur because strengths are "used up" by the time individuals enter treatment, so that differences in variables indicating various past skills and psychological abilities are moot.

As column 2 suggests, the various findings generally remain when controlling for response bias. The major change is that the coefficient attached to the baseline measure of use of controlled substances gains statistical significance.

Mediation. According to previous analyses, both interventions increase the dollars subjects receive from income maintenance agencies at the time of the first follow-up interview, although the case management only services lead to the greater increment. Both also improved use of employment-related services at this time.[10] The relations suggest that the services follow the intended model and stress provision of access to tangible support. In keeping with the model, it was hypothesized that such access to benefits and employment services would improve later residential stability (by improving access to income).

As summarized in column 3, reported receipt of income maintenance grants at the first follow-up interview indeed predicts residential stability at the second such interview. However, the use of employment counseling at the first follow-up interview is not predictive. This latter finding is paralleled by analyses (not reported here) suggesting that the interventions did not have an impact on the number of days subjects worked at the time of the second follow-up interview. Apparently, attempts to improve work readiness were not successful.

The coefficients attached to the interventions lose statistical significance when including the mediating variables. In total, results thus suggest that the impact of the interventions on later residential stability is largely attributable to the ability of workers to help subjects obtain income maintenance support during the course of treatment. Although this is not reported in a table, further analysis suggests that the impact of this mediating factor is reduced to statistical insignificance when adding a measure of residential stability at the first follow-up interview; the coefficients attached to the two interventions also fail to predict the criterion variable in this equation. The major effect of receipt of income maintenance benefits at the first follow-up interview thus may be to improve housing stability at the time clients exit treatment. Apparently, the improvement is sustained at the second follow-up interview.

The correction for sample bias, which is reported in column 4 of Table 3, confirms the impact of reported receipt of income maintenance benefits. However, the coefficient attached to the case management only intervention regains statistical significance. This implies that receipt of income maintenance at the time the intervention is ended is not the only reason for the impact of the case management only intervention. Perhaps housing stability is also partly achieved by the direct efforts workers undertake to help individuals look for housing. (The measure of combined alcohol and drug use at the baseline, which falls barely short of statistical significance in the uncorrected equation, also becomes a significant predictor in this model.)

DISCUSSION

The analyses provide evidence that both interventions reduce substance abuse while they increase residential stability one year after program enrollment. While efficacy seems modest for the prediction of substance abuse, it is nevertheless noteworthy when considering that members of the control group improved markedly. In comparative terms, the reduction in substance abuse by members of the case management only intervention is 45% of the mean score on the variable; the improvement in residential stability is also relatively large. While the intervention model needs further tests within populations in which the control group does not improve as dramatically, it seems reasonably efficacious in the current context.

To be sure, the finding that the case management only intervention is of equal or greater effectiveness as the housing intervention is at some odds with previous suggestions that homelessness is largely a housing problem.[3] The finding may indicate that case management services are primary, and as has been mentioned, that clients in the housing group benefit less from certain of the more tangible community services. However, while the value of the less expensive case management only intervention is highlighted by these results, it must be considered that the housing intervention has a higher acceptance rate and thus reached a larger proportion of approached adults.

The analyses of reasons for impact give some credence to the progressive independence model's premise that change may be brought about by interventions aimed at meeting multiple concerns. That is, impact of the interventions on substance abuse apparently occurs partly because the interventions improve the utilization of outpatient substance abuse services during treatment. We tentatively attribute the improved outcome to the value of services, or to the increased motivation caused by attendance at treatment sessions. In turn, we attribute the increased utilization to the resources offered by the interventions; individuals might agree to remain in treatment because participation is required to obtain the tangible help the program has to offer, and because tangible needs are met to a sufficient degree to enable clients to focus on recovery.

A reduction in avoidance coping is also implicated in improved abstinence. The impact may occur because individuals learn to confront problems that lead to relapses. The improved coping style, in turn, may reflect the use of the cognitive behavioral relapse prevention model.

Subjects in part improve residential stability due to their receipt of income maintenance benefits at the time of the intervention, which is attributable to the advocacy of workers for this needed source of funds for housing. This is a promising finding in the sense that it suggests that workers who focus on tangible concerns can help reduce the homelessness of their clients. As previously noted, direct advocacy for housing may also be implicated for clients in the case management only intervention. However, the results also indicate the dependence of the population on welfare benefits; while the majority of sample members have a reasonable work history, the interventions did not demonstrate the ability to improve employment opportunities. This occurs even though subjects increased their use of employment services. Perhaps the subjects' history of abuse, limited education, race, and lack of recent work limit opportunities. One general point may be that a community-oriented intervention depends for its success on the resources available to a given population in a given locale at a given time.

CONCLUSION

Results most generally suggest that the services offered by the progressive independence model help reduce substance abuse and homelessness among members of this sample. In light of the presumed difficulties encountered by the interventions cited in the introduction, this seems to be an important result. But it is particularly notable that the current treatment model pays attention to short-term tangible needs first, and also combines help for abuse, other personal problems, and long-term financial needs. Indeed, results concerning mediating variables suggest that the provision of tangible aid, as well as various aspects of the counseling program, lead to the positive outcomes. Therefore, despite previous thoughts that this would be difficult, the analysis also provides some evidence that there is a generally efficacious way of combining the remediation of tangible, long-term financial, and substance abuse problems. These findings, combined with the apparent ineffectiveness of traditional approaches, support the conclusion that interventions aimed at substance abuse and homelessness should place a higher priority on meeting multiple needs.

NOTES

1. Sosin MR. Homeless and vulnerable meal program users: A comparison study. Social Problems. 1992; 39:170-88.

2. Piliavin I, Sosin MR, Westerfelt H. Explaining long-term homelessness. Social Service Review. 1993; 4:576-98.

3. Roth D, Bean J. Alcohol problems and homelessness: Findings from the Ohio study. Presented at the National Institute on Alcoholism and Alcohol Abuse, "The homeless with alcohol related problems," special meeting, 1985.

4. Fischer PJ, Breakey W. Profile of the Baltimore homeless with alcohol problems. Alcohol Health and Research World. 1987; 11:36-7.

5. Welte JW, Barnes GM. Drinking among homeless and marginally housed adults in New York state. J Stud Alcohol. 1992; 53:303-15.

6. Koegel P, Burnham MA. Traditional and non-traditional homeless alcoholics. Alcohol Health and Research World. 1987; 11:28-33.

7. Bahr H, Caplow T. Old men drunk and sober. New York: New York University Press, 1974.

8. Blumberg L, Shipley TE, Shandler IW. Skid row and its alternatives. Philadelphia: Temple University Press, 1973.

9. Grigsby C, Baumann, D, Gregorich SE, Roberts-Gray C. Disaffiliation to entrenchment: A model for understanding homelessness. Journal of Social Issues. 1990; 46:141-156.

10. Sosin MR, Yamaguchi J, Bruni M, Grossman S, Leonelli B, Reidy M, Schwingen J. Treating homelessness and substance abuse in community context: A case management and supported housing demonstration. Chicago: School of Social Service Administration, University of Chicago, 1994.

11. Sosin MR, Schwingen J, Yamaguchi J. Case management and supported housing in Chicago: The interaction of program resources and client characteristics. Alcoholism Treatment Quarterly. 1993; 10:35-50.

12. Sosin MR, Yamaguchi J. Case management routines and discretion in a program addressing homelessness and substance abuse (submitted).

13. Moos RH, Finney JW. The expanding scope of alcoholism treatment evaluation. Am Psychol. 1983; 38:1035-44.

14. Bromet EJ, Moos R. Environmental resources and the post-treatment functioning of alcoholic patients. J Health Soc Behav. 1977; 18:326-35.

15. Marlatt GA, Gordon JR (eds.). Relapse prevention: Maintenance strategies in the treatment of addictive behaviors. New York: Guilford Press, 1985.

16. Stark MJ. Dropping out of substance abuse treatment: A clinically oriented review. Clinical Psychology Review. 1992; 12:93-116.

17. Breakey W. Treating the homeless. Alcohol Health and Research World. 1987; 11:42-47.

18. Shipley T, Shandler I, Penn M. Treatment and research with homeless alcoholics. Contemporary Drug Problems. 1989; Fall, 505-26.

19. Sosin MR, Colson P, Grossman S. Homelessness in Chicago: Poverty and pathology, social institutions and social change. Chicago: Chicago Community Trust and School of Social Service Administration, The University of Chicago, 1988.

20. Brown BB. Social and psychological correlates of help-seeking behavior among urban adults. Am J Community Psychol. 1978; 6:425-39.

21. Colson P. Service use among the homeless. Doctoral dissertation, The University of Chicago, The School of Social Service Administration, 1990.

22. McLellan AT, Kushner H, Metzger D, Peters R, Smith I, Grissom G, Pettinati H and Argeriou M. The fifth edition of the Addiction Severity Index: Historical critique and normative data. J Subst Abuse Treat. 1992.

23. Jaccard J, Turrisi R, Wan CK. Interaction effects in multiple regression. Newbury Park, CA: Sage Publications, 1990.

24. Heckman J. Sample selection bias as a specification error. Econometrica. 1979; 47:153-61.

25. Huppert FA, Walters DE, Nicholas ED, Elliott BJ. The factor structure of the General Health Questionnaire (GHQ-30). Br J Psychiatry. 1989; 155:178-85.

26. Littrell J. Understanding and treating alcoholism. Hillsdale, NJ: Lawrence Erlbaum Associates, 1991.

27. Baekeland F, Lundwall, L. Dropping out of treatment: A critical review. Psychol Bull. 1977; 82:738-83.

28. Simpson DD. Treatment for drug abuse: Follow-up outcomes and length of time spent. Arch Gen Psychiatry. 1981; 38:875-80.

Assessing the Value
of a Short-Term Residential Drug
Treatment Program
for Homeless Men

Julie A. Lam, PhD
James F. Jekel, MD
Kenneth S. Thompson, MD
Philip J. Leaf, PhD
Stephanie W. Hartwell, PhD
Lou Florio, MS

Julie A. Lam is affiliated with the Northeast Program Evaluation Center/182, VA Medical Center, West Haven, CT 06516.

James F. Jekel if affiliated with the Department of Epidemiology and Public Health, Yale University School of Medicine, New Haven, CT 06510.

Kenneth S. Thompson is affiliated with the Division of Public Psychiatry Western Psychiatric Institute and Clinic, University of Pittsburgh Medical Center, Pittsburgh, PA 15213.

Philip J. Leaf is affiliated with the Department of Mental Hygiene, Johns Hopkins University, Baltimore, MD 21205.

Stephanie W. Hartwell is affiliated with the Connecticut Department of Mental Health, 500 Vine Street, Hartford, CT 06112.

Lou Florio is affiliated with the Department of Epidemiology and Public Health, Yale University School of Medicine, New Haven, CT 06510.

Address correspondence to James F. Jekel, MD, Department of Epidemiology and Public Health, Yale University School of Medicine, 60 College Street, New Haven, CT 06510.

This project was funded by the National Institute on Alcohol Abuse and Alcoholism (5 U01 AA08774-03) in consultation with the National Institute on Drug Abuse. An earlier version of this paper was presented at the 1994 meeting of the American Public Health Association.

[Haworth co-indexing entry note]: "Assessing the Value of a Short-Term Residential Drug Treatment Program for Homeless Men." Lam, Julie A. et al. Co-published simultaneously in the *Journal of Addictive Diseases* (The Haworth Medical Press, an imprint of The Haworth Press, Inc.) Vol. 14, No. 4, 1995, pp. 21-39; and: *The Effectiveness of Social Interventions for Homeless Substance Abusers* (ed: Gerald J. Stahler) The Haworth Medical Press, an imprint of The Haworth Press, Inc., 1995, pp. 21-39. Single or multiple copies of this article are available from The Haworth Document Delivery Service [1-800-342-9678; 9:00 a.m. - 5:00 p.m. (EST)].

SUMMARY. Cocaine and other substance abuse has been found to be a contributing or primary cause of homelessness in urban men. This project evaluated the effectiveness of the Grant Street Partnership (GSP), a shelter-based treatment program for homeless, cocaine-abusing men, consisting of 90 days of residential treatment and 6 months of aftercare. We tested the hypothesis that the 182 men randomized to the GSP group, as compared to the 112 men randomized to a "usual services" group, would show significantly greater improvement over time in the areas of drug use and residential and economic stability. An 80% response rate was achieved overall for the five follow-up points. *Cocaine use,* defined as use of cocaine at least once in the prior 30 days, declined from about 90% at baseline for both groups to 11% in the GSP group and 55% in the control group at 21 months. The GSP group was also more likely than the usual services group to have achieved *residential stability* by the time of the 9 month follow-up. Neither group experienced an improvement over time in *employment status. [Article copies available from The Haworth Document Delivery Service: 1-800-342-9678.]*

INTRODUCTION

The Grant Street Partnership (GSP) was a short-term shelter and day treatment program designed to rehabilitate homeless, cocaine-abusing men in New Haven, CT. It was created as part of a large multi-site collaborative research-demonstration project administered by the National Institute of Alcohol Abuse and Alcoholism (NIAAA).[1]

The relationship between illegal drug abuse and homelessness has not been studied thoroughly. For example, a 1991 publication of the Alcohol, Drug Abuse, and Mental Health administration stated that, "Compared to investigations of mental illness and alcoholism in the contemporary homeless population, little effort has been expended on examining patterns of abuse of drugs other than alcohol."[2] The GSP represented one of the first attempts nationally to address specifically the special complex of problems common to homeless users of cocaine, a problem that co-occurs frequently with alcohol and other drug abuse. For example, Spinner and Leaf surveyed 181 persons in the five emergency shelters in New Haven during a four-week interval in November and December of 1990. They found that, in the 30 days before the interview, 53% of the respondents had used alcohol to intoxication, 41% had used cocaine, and 27% had used marijuana. Two thirds of the respondents identified substance use as a reason for their homelessness, and approximately one third of the shelter respondents reported drug-related criminal activity.[3]

The GSP was created to achieve three related goals: (1) reduction of substance abuse, particularly cocaine; (2) promotion of more stable living situations; and (3) improved economic and employment status. These changes were to be achieved through: provision of a drug-free, modified therapeutic community consisting of 90 days of residential care and 6 months of after-care case management; the phased resumption of responsibilities; and the provision of relapse prevention skills. Through group therapy, a specific service plan, and other kinds of assistance and support, the program sought to foster empowerment, self-determination, and the enhancement of daily living skills, drug-free survival skills, and community living skills. The program was designed only for men, because there was no possibility of making separate dormitories for men and women, and there were no facilities for children of the women.[1]

The GSP was a new program, with both the building and the program designed specifically to serve the target group. The 90-day residential shelter was located in a former factory building, with the first floor remodeled for the GSP. The building was in the shape of an L, with one arm being the dormitory, the reception/office area at the bend, and the areas for meetings, exercise, art, education, dining room, and kitchen being in the other arm. Beds were in cubicles separated by partitions but open to the center walkway. Each resident has his own locker for his personal possessions.

The program consisted of three progress levels. Men started in the lowest (Orientation) level, in which they had essentially no privileges outside the shelter, but had a "big brother" to help them adapt and understand the process. In this level a man's time was devoted to meetings with his case manager, development of a plan for his treatment in the GSP and beyond, daily therapeutic group meetings (some of which were in-house AA/NA meetings), and individual counseling.

As a resident progressed to the second (Resource Implementation) level, he could become a big brother to an incoming resident; he could use the telephone and could travel to outside events if accompanied. He continued working with his case manager, especially focusing on housing and employment. He continued to meet with the psychosocial counselor, with group psychoeducational sessions, and with AA/NA meetings in the facility or, occasionally now, outside the facility. If his record was good, he could also get 6-hour passes every other week.

In the top (Re-entry) level, a resident developed a continuing plan for housing, education, and employment, and even starting education or employment commitments. He was required to open a savings account and to develop an aftercare plan for when he was discharged. He continued in regular meetings, as above.

The 6 months of aftercare was to focus on housing, employment, skill-building, and improving relationships. This was to have consisted of weekly meetings for the first two months, augmented with meetings with the client's family, job counselor, and others. After the first two months, these meetings were to be less often, but at least biweekly. Although there was some contact with many of the graduates after they left, this was mostly initiated by the clients and took place at the GSP. A frequent change in personnel in the case management unit meant that ties were frequently broken, and the case managers were frequently shorthanded. Thus the aftercare program varied between weak and non-existent, depending on the time and the client.

The existing homeless and substance abuse services in New Haven (here called "usual services") were fairly extensive. All of the several homeless shelters had case workers who sought to counsel the men into appropriate services and programs, including drug treatment and vocational training programs. There were several drug abuse treatment programs in New Haven, but they usually had waiting lists of 3 months or longer. Needed medical care was available at both of the city's hospitals, as well as at neighborhood health centers. Numerous AA/NA programs were available.

RESEARCH DESIGN AND METHODS

This research project included both an outcome and a process evaluation of the GSP. Quantitative and qualitative methods were used to collect data for both phases of the evaluation. This paper describes the design of the outcome evaluation and focuses on the quantitative results of that evaluation.

The outcome evaluation employed an experimental design in which eligible men were detoxed, given a baseline interview, and then randomized either to the treatment (GSP) or control (usual community services) condition. Subjects in both groups were then followed and interviewed at three, six, nine, 15, and 21 months post-baseline. The interviews used structured questionnaires consisting of the core instruments: Personal History Form (PHF); Addiction Severity Index (ASI); and Treatment Services Interview (TSI) (at follow-up), as well as a number of site-specific items.

The total number of men completing baseline interviews was 294 (GSP group = 182, usual services group = 112). The numbers in the two groups were unequal because early in the GSP program, randomization had to be suspended for four months to enable a critical mass of residents to build up so there would be enough people in the program to make it attractive. The suspension of randomization did not adversely affect the similarity of the GSP and control groups, but it did decrease the number of men in the usual services (control) group considerably, especially those eligible for the later interviews, and thereby compromised the study's power to detect all but very large improvements in the 15 and 21 month interviews.

Funding for the project ended prior to the completion of all of the 9, 15, and 21 month interviews, so that many of the men were not yet eligible for the later interviews, because they had not been in the program long enough. Nine month interviews were completed by 237 of the men (81% of all and 86% of those who were eligible); 150 completed the 15 month interview (51% of all, and 89% of those who were eligible), and 69 completed the 21 month interview (23% of all but 90% of those who were eligible).

The overall response rate for the project was 80% of those eligible for a given interview. This rate reflects the relatively low response rate for the three and six month interviews, particularly in the control group. The lowest response rate observed in either group in any interview was in the three month interviews for the control group (64%). This was the only point at which the control and treatment groups differed significantly in their follow-up completion rates, and the low response rate was due to the fact that many of the men in the control group, not being in an organized program, were initially lost to follow-up. However, special efforts resulted in the study's finding most of them for subsequent interviews.

As with all research in which study groups are followed over time, losses (either losses to follow-up or censorship because a study ended before subjects reached the full duration of follow-up) reduced the numbers (and hence the power). Incomplete follow-up also raises the possibility of selection bias. In such a circumstance, the best protection is a high follow-up rate for those who are eligible for data collection. In the New Haven study, the follow-up rates for eligible residents were high for the 9, 15 and 21 month interviews. The overall follow-up rates were similar for those interviews for which men were eligible. For example, overall 82% of the eligible GSP group interviews occurred, vs. 78% for the control group. For the 9 month interviews, 87% of the eligible men in the GSP were interviewed vs. 85% in the control group. The comparable figures for the 15 month interviews were 86% vs. 97%, and for the 21 month interviews these figures were 90% vs. 92%. Similarly, 75% of interviews for which whites were eligible were obtained, compared to 85% for blacks, and 74% for Latinos.

Because study subjects were admitted over time, there is the possibility of a cohort effect. We could not study that, because the later entrants did not have their final interviews, but we know of no reason the early entrants should differ greatly from those who entered later. A systematic change over time in the characteristics of the men could bias our findings, particularly the 15 and 21 month interviews.

A more serious problem was the fact that only about one third of the GSP residents stayed the full 90 days and graduated. Many others stayed almost to that time but left or acted out and were dismissed within the last two weeks. Moreover, particularly until the program got clearly established, some of the men would start the program but find there were not enough other men in the program for them to feel comfortable, and would leave. Analyses showed that those men who stayed for the full 90 days consistently did better on the primary outcome variables than those who left early, but this cannot be considered solid evidence of program effectiveness. The length of stay may only have been an index for other client variables, such as motivation for change, and may not, therefore, be a reliable index of program effectiveness.

RESULTS

The experimental and control groups were compared on 60 variables to determine the equivalence of the two study groups at baseline. Categorical variables were compared using chi-square, Fisher's exact probability test, or risk ratio with Cornfield's method for calculating the confidence intervals in the EPIINFO computer package.[4] Continuous variables were tested using t-tests or one-way ANOVAs. Alpha was set in advance at 0.05.

Five of the 60 variables (6.7%) showed statistically significant differences, which is about what would have been expected by chance. The differences at baseline included the GSP group showing a higher total income, due mainly to more illegal income, and a lower percent admitting to the purchase of cocaine (65% vs. 90%). Also, a higher proportion of GSP subjects had used heroin in the previous 30 days (35% vs. 21%) and had ever received drug treatment (79% vs. 66%). The experimental and usual services (control) groups had very similar follow-up rates–in the high 80% range for the interview times focused on for this analysis (9, 15, and 21 months).

Demographic Characteristics
of the Study Population at Baseline

Table 1 summarizes the demographic and background characteristics of the study population. The average age of the men in the New Haven study

TABLE 1. Demographic and Social Characteristics of the Study Population at Baseline by Group.

Variable	GSP	Control	Total
Sample Size	(182)	(112)	(294)
Age (mean years)	32.6	32.5	32.5
(S.D.)	6.8	7.5	7.1
Race			
White	20.9	24.1	22.1
Black	57.1	61.6	58.8
Latino	22.0	13.4	18.7
Education (mean years)	11.4	11.4	11.4
(S.D.)	2.1	1.9	2.0
Income (all sources—$)	1029.45	771.54*	931.11
(S.D.)	1592.74	885.74	1371.16
Marital status			
Married	7.7	8.0	7.8
Remarried	0.0	0.0	0.0
Widow	1.6	0.0	1.0
Separated	14.3	13.4	13.9
Divorced	18.7	14.3	17.0
Never Married	57.7	64.3	60.2
Parental status			
(% with Children)	61.5	67.0	63.6
Mean # of Children	1.5	1.5	1.5

*$p < 0.05$ **$p < 0.01$

was 32.5 years. The majority of the men were African-American, with approximately equal numbers of whites and Latinos (mostly from Puerto Rico). The average number of years of education completed was 11.4, with nearly 40 percent of the men not completing high school. The majority of the men were never married, while nearly two thirds of the men had children.

Reduction of Cocaine and Other Substance Abuse

The primary goal of the GSP was to reduce substance abuse among its mostly cocaine-abusing client population. Table 2 gives an overall picture of the substance use patterns of the two groups and of the total sample at baseline and at 9, 15, and 21 months following randomization.

The use of cocaine decreased dramatically in both the GSP and control groups. Table 2 shows that at the 9 month follow-up, 31.2% of the men overall had used cocaine at least once in the previous 30 days, compared with 89.1% at the time of the baseline interview. There was a further reduction in the percentage of men using cocaine at the 15 and 21 month interviews. By 21 months, the GSP group had continued to decline in their use of cocaine, but the control group men had *increased* their cocaine use.

Similarly, the use of alcohol also decreased over time for both groups. Marijuana and heroin use showed similar, though less dramatic, patterns of decline. Multi-substance use also decreased dramatically from baseline, and the GSP group was significantly less likely to be abusing poly-substances at the 9 month interview (p = 0.02). Composite scores were calculated for each of the drug and alcohol domains of the ASI.[5] The composite scores combine a number of variables measuring aspects of each domain, and a higher score is less desirable. There were no significant differences between the groups in drug or alcohol composite scores at any of the follow-up points.

Multiple regression was used to find variables strongly associated with continued cocaine use in the total study group (i.e., both GSP and Control men). In the multivariable analyses, the variable designating the group (GSP = 1, Control = 0) was always entered. We focused on the nine month follow-up point for the regression analysis because most of the research subjects were enrolled in the project long enough to be eligible for a nine month interview.

Panel A of Table 3 shows a four variable model that explained 42% of the variance in cocaine use during the past 30 days at the 9 month interview. The variable most strongly associated with cocaine use was involvement in illegal activities to make money. As can be assumed given the high financial cost of drug addiction, men who were using cocaine were more

TABLE 2. Substance abuse patterns at baseline, 9, 15, and 21 months.

Sample sizes

Interview	Grant St.	Control	Total
	N	N	N
Baseline	182	112	294
9 Month	148	89	237
15 Month	104	46	150
21 Month	52	17	69

Percent using cocaine last 30 days

Interview	Grant St.	Control	Total
Baseline	89.0	89.3	89.1
9 month	27.7	37.1	31.2
15 month	28.8	23.9	27.3
21 month	21.2	41.2	26.1

Percent using alcohol last 30 days

Interview	Grant St.	Control	Total
Baseline	80.8	75.0	78.6
9 month	38.5	48.3	42.2
15 month	37.5	39.1	38.0
21 month	32.7	47.1	36.2

Percent using more than one substance per day last 30 days

Interview	Grant St.	Control	Total
Baseline	82.3	81.1	81.9
9 month	25.0	39.3*	30.4
15 month	28.8	28.3	28.7
21 month	21.2	29.4	23.2

*p < 0.05   **p < 0.01

TABLE 2 (continued)

DRUG COMPOSITE SCORE

Interview	Grant St.		Control		Total	
	Mean	STD	Mean	STD	Mean	STD
Baseline	0.38	0.18	0.36	0.17	0.37	0.17
9 month	0.09	0.11	0.08	0.09	0.08	0.10
15 month	0.08	0.11	0.06	0.10	0.08	0.11
21 month	0.06	0.09	0.07	0.09	0.06	0.09

ALCOHOL COMPOSITE SCORE

Interview	Grant St.		Control		Total	
	Mean	STD	Mean	STD	Mean	STD
Baseline	0.34	0.33	0.32	0.33	0.33	0.33
9 month	0.10	0.17	0.15	0.21	0.12	0.19
15 month	0.12	0.21	0.12	0.21	0.12	0.21
21 month	0.07	0.20	0.12	0.23	0.08	0.21

$^*p < 0.05$ $^{**}p < 0.01$

likely to be involved in illegal money-making activities (i.e., selling illegal drugs). Other significant variables were the use of substance abuse treatment services at any time during the 60 days prior to the interview, age, and the proportion of one's life spent using cocaine (log transformations were used here to normalize skewed distributions). Men who had engaged in some type of treatment over the past two months were less likely to be using cocaine. The older the subject, the more likely he was to be using cocaine, but also the greater the proportion of a man's life he had used cocaine, the less likely he was to be using cocaine at the 9 month interview.

Increase in Residential Stability

A second goal of the GSP was to increase the residential stability of the participants. The men in this study were not the traditional chronically homeless. The average study participant first became homeless at age 28 and had been homeless three times in his life. By far, the most often mentioned reason (multiple reasons could be given) for first becoming homeless was

TABLE 3. Stepwise regression results–maximum R-square improvement.

Panel A: Dependent variable is number of days of cocaine use in the past 30 days–9 mo. interview

Variable Entered	Associated with	Cumulative R-Square	p-value
Money from illegal activities	More days cocaine use	.33	.0001
Days of treatment/subs. abuse	Fewer days cocaine use	.38	.0001
Age	More days cocaine use	.40	.003
Proportion life using cocaine	Fewer days cocaine use	.42	.01
REGRESSION		.42	.0001

Panel B: Dependent variable is number of days literally homeless in the past 30 days–9 mo. interview

Variable Entered	Associated with	Cumulative R-Square	p-value
Grant St. Partnership group	Fewer days literally homeless	.04	.005
Black study participant	More days literally homeless	.06	.04
Proportion of life using coke	Fewer days literally homeless	.08	.05
REGRESSION		.08	.004

Panel C: Dependent variable is number of days worked for pay in the past 30 days–9 mo. interview

Variable Entered	Associated with	Cumulative R-Square	p-value
Intravenous drug use	Fewer days worked	.04	.0003
History of family subs. use	More days worked	.07	.006
Use of marijuana	Fewer days worked	.11	.002
Income at baseline	Fewer days worked	.12	.058
(Ln) Number of substance abuse treatment visits	Fewer days worked	.14	.006
(Ln) Total number of visits for services	More days worked	.15	.02
REGRESSION		.15	.0001

alcohol or drug problems; this was followed by interpersonal conflict–such as separation, divorce, or arguments–and that the people with whom the respondent was living made him leave.

Table 4 shows the men's residential patterns at baseline, 9, 15, and 21 months. Housing status can be conceptualized as falling into four categories: (1) literally homeless (e.g., sleeping in indoor or outdoor public places, cars, emergency shelters, or in crack or base houses); (2) marginally housed

TABLE 4. Housing stability at baseline, 9, 15, and 21 months.

Interview	Grant Street	Control	Total
PERCENT LITERALLY HOMELESS FOR 1+ DAYS IN LAST 60			
Baseline %	72.5	77.7	74.5
9 mo. %	13.5	28.1**	19.0
15 mo. %	13.5	15.2	14.0
21 mo. %	7.7	5.9	7.3
PERCENT MARGINALLY HOMELESS FOR 1+ DAYS IN LAST 60			
Baseline %	50.0	57.1	52.7
9 mo. %	25.7	44.9**	32.9
15 mo. %	26.0	30.4	27.3
21 mo. %	30.8	41.2	33.3
PERCENT INSTITUTIONALLY HOUSED FOR 1+ DAY IN LAST 60			
Baseline %	27.5	30.4	28.6
9 mo. %	34.5	38.2	35.9
15 mo. %	35.6	30.4	34.0
21 mo. %	38.5	29.4	36.2
PERCENT TRADITIONALLY HOUSED FOR 1+ DAY IN LAST 60			
Baseline %	42.9	38.4	41.2
9 mo. %	62.2	56.2	59.9
15 mo. %	64.4	63.0	64.0
21 mo. %	63.5	58.8	62.3

$*p < 0.05$ $**p < 0.01$

(e.g., hotel/motel, someone else's place, or transitional housing; (3) institutional (e.g., hospital or treatment program, jail, prison, or corrections halfway house; and (4) traditionally or stably housed (e.g., own SRO room, apartment or house, boarding house or board and care facility, group home, long-term alcohol and drug-free facility, or parent/guardian's apartment or house).

Overall, the percentage of those who were literally homeless decreased steadily over time. Also, for the men who spent some days literally homeless, the average number of days out of the past 60 spent that way declined sharply from 23 at baseline to 2 at 21 months. The GSP group was consistently less likely to be literally homeless, although the difference was statistically significant only at 9 months post-randomization (p = 0.006).

The proportion of study subjects who were marginally homeless declined from baseline to 9 months, but it began increasing after that, although it never reached the level it was at baseline. The average number of days marginally homeless dropped at 9 months but then returned to the baseline level and stayed there. The GSP group was consistently less likely to be marginally homeless, but the difference was statistically significant only at 9 months.

The proportion of subjects who were institutionalized remained stable over time. Between 29% and 36% of the men were institutionalized at each of the assessment points. The percentage of men who spent at least one night traditionally housed increased by about 21 percentage points from baseline to 21 month follow-up. The average number of days the men were traditionally housed out of the previous 60 days increased from 14 days at baseline to 33 days at the 21 month interview.

Table 3, Panel B shows the three variable model that was arrived at to explain the number of days spent literally homeless during the past 60 at the time of the 9 month interview. However, this model only accounted for 8% of the variance in homelessness. Men assigned to the GSP group were less likely to have spent time literally homeless over the past 60 days. *As with cocaine use, men who had spent more of their lives using cocaine were less likely to be literally homeless.* Compared to the deleted category, whites, (race was entered as dummied variables) blacks were more likely to be literally homeless at the 9 month interview.

Enhancement of Economic and Employment Status

The third goal of the GSP was to encourage advancement in education and employment opportunities for the participants. Table 5 represents the economic situation of the study participants at baseline, 9, 15, and 21 months.

Overall, the employment status of the study population improved only a

TABLE 5. Employment status at baseline, 9, 15, and 21 months.

Interview	GSP	Control	Total
Mean number of days worked in last 30 days			
Baseline	3.5	3.7	3.6
9 month	9.7	10.1	8.9
15 month	8.7	9.5	8.9
21 month	7.6	5.6	7.1
Percent who worked in last 30 days			
Baseline	32.6	32.1	32.4
9 month	56.1	55.1	55.7
15 month	48.5	52.2	49.7
21 month	42.3	37.5	41.2
Mean income from all sources in last 30 days			
Baseline	1029.45	771.54*	931.11
9 month	941.90	738.90	865.70
15 month	857.10	756.60	826.30
21 month	899.80	727.50	857.30
Mean income from:			
a. Employment			
Baseline	166.00	182.20	172.17
9 month	337.90	358.10	345.50
15 month	309.50	349.50	321.80
21 month	380.40	128.60*	317.50
b. Public assistance			
Baseline	90.80	104.60	96.08
9 month	112.90	100.20	108.20
15 month	113.40	114.70	113.80
21 month	87.50	176.10*	108.30

Interview	GSP	Control	Total
c. Mate/family/friends			
Baseline	49.92	51.62	50.57
9 month	25.70	52.10	35.60
15 month	34.40	24.30	31.30
21 month	30.00	54.40	36.00
d. Illegal sources			
Baseline	663.41	355.40	546.30
9 month	306.00	78.40*	220.20
15 month	244.70	100.00	200.70
21 month	255.50	182.40	237.50

*$p < 0.05$ **$p < 0.01$

small amount when measured by the number of days worked for pay out of the previous 30. Table 6 shows that from baseline to 21 months, the mean number of days working increased only from a mean of 3.6 days to 7.1 days. The percentage of men who worked at least one day in the past 30 also increased, although not dramatically, from 32% at baseline to about 53% at 9 months and back down to 41% at 21 months. The two groups did not differ significantly at any follow-up point in either the proportion who worked or the number of days worked.

The total monthly income of the men in both groups changed little over time as well. However, looking at income from all sources combined ignores where the men were obtaining their money. Over time, the percentage of men receiving income from public assistance declined, those receiving income from legitimate employment increased at 9 months and then declined slowly; those receiving money from family and friends remained about the same; and the percentage of men making money illegally also dropped. Men in the GSP group received significantly less income from public assistance than those in the Control group at the time of the 21 month interview, and more income from legitimate employment. The GSP group also received less money from family and friends.

We also compared composite scores for employment status over time. The employment status composite included items measuring work and income patterns and needs. As might be expected from the discussion of the individual variables, the composite score for the total group improved only slightly, from .82 at baseline to .76 at the 21 month interview.

Multiple regression results revealed a six variable model explaining 15% of the variance in the number of days worked for pay in the past 30 at the 9 month interview (see Table 3, Panel C). Not surprisingly, men who were using illegal drugs, either intravenous drugs or marijuana, or who were receiving substance abuse treatment, worked fewer days than those who did not. Family history of substance abuse, however, was positively related to working, indicating that those with family histories of substance abuse were *more* likely to be working. This finding was unexpected, and the explanation is unclear. The use of all services was positively related to employment, indicating that the more total services a subject used the more likely he was to be working; some of these services may have been employment assistance. Finally, the amount of total income was positively related to the days worked for pay; this was probably due to the income from employment.

DISCUSSION

The GSP had a positive impact on its participants in at least two ways: (1) their cocaine use decreased, and they were more likely than the control group to maintain their abstinence with the passage of time; and (2) they were somewhat more likely at 9 months to be living in stable housing arrangements, although differences between the groups became smaller with the passage of time.

Of major interest was the fact that in most areas *except for employment*, there was an impressive improvement in *both* the intervention and control groups. We suggest three possible explanations for this improvement. First, it is possible that at baseline, problems were exaggerated by the study subjects in an attempt to get into the program. Second, by virtue of their seeking the program, most of the study subjects in both groups were presenting themselves for change, so presumably they had come to a point in their lives where they wanted things to go differently, and they made that happen. Third, and very important from our perspective, this could be an example of regression toward the mean, which is frequently-seen in programs where those people with the most severe problems are given priority for admission. By selecting subjects at their worst, they have nowhere to go but up, and they may have been able to organize themselves and their resources to improve. Given *time* and any kind of *help* (special or usual services), the study subjects were able to make progress in those areas in which they had the greatest influence, namely substance abuse and housing. However, despite the overall improvement of both groups, the GSP group generally improved more than did the control group subjects.

It was not surprising that little improvement occurred in employment. Improvement in employability is a long-term process requiring the improvement of both skills and attitudes. Moreover, actual employment is heavily dependent on the availability of jobs for which the study subjects have skills, and on the quality of the community system for putting potential workers and jobs together. Both of these factors were deficient in New Haven.

We also found that the variables most closely associated with "doing well" or what could be called proxies for success were: (1) not being involved in *illegal activities,* (2) continuing in some type of *substance abuse treatment,* and, to a lesser extent, (3) being in the *GSP group*. Each of these represents ways in which individuals structured time. Illegal activities structure time in such a way that drug use is an integral part of that time. Substance abuse treatment (attending NA/AA meetings and the like) and being a part of the GSP structure time in another, more positive, way. Jobs would be another manner of filling time for these men, but one that is not readily available to them in New Haven at this time. The results of our evaluation suggest that finding ways to positively structure their time leads to less drug use and more stable lives and living situations for the homeless men in our study.

One somewhat surprising finding was that the more a man had used cocaine throughout his life, the less likely he was to be using cocaine at the 9 month interview. This may support the argument often heard from the men in the study that you have to "hit bottom" completely before you can even think about giving up crack cocaine. In other words, it is not necessarily age that determines whether a man has had enough, but how long and hard he has used cocaine, regardless of age.

CONCLUSION

For practical purposes, the GSP was only a short-term (90-day) residential drug treatment program, because the six months of continuing case management services (the "aftercare program") was never really implemented. It is somewhat encouraging, however, that despite the relatively short duration of treatment, the basic comparison of all GSP group members with all control group members revealed positive, although modest, results. There was an indication from the 21 month interviews completed that members of the GSP group were better able than control group members to maintain their abstinence over the long run (at least 21 months). Only longer term follow-up would determine if this trend holds.

Cocaine addiction and homelessness were the most immediate problems the men faced. Nevertheless, there was a panoply of other problems: cross addiction to opiates and alcohol; long-standing poverty; a recent personal crisis; a profound sense of demoralization, cynicism, and powerlessness; cultural alienation and entrapment in an often brutal "street culture"; unemployment; undereducation; histories of criminality and violence contemporaneous with histories of trauma, exploitation, and victimization; troubled interpersonal relations; distressed and disorganized families with few resources; legal problems; medical illnesses, including HIV infection; and psychiatric comorbidities, including a disturbed sense of self and others which would likely be manifested in help-rejection, denial, and manipulativeness. Homelessness and addiction constituted a particular channel into which these men had fallen, both due to their own propensity and to the instability of the social margin in which they had grown up and which they and their families continued to inhabit. Many of the men had hit bottom and were ready to make changes in their lives when they entered our research project, as evidenced by the generally positive trends in substance use and residential stability for both groups. Above and beyond that, however, the treatment and case management services the men received from the GSP made positive inroads into breaking their cycle of cocaine abuse and homelessness. Their time was structured in a productive manner while in the program and many of the men continued to find positive ways of structuring their time upon their departure.

Although this study provides modest support for programs of the GSP type, it also indicates that it would be erroneous to consider "usual services" to be of no value. When men such as these have hit bottom and are ready for change, they may be able to profit from any help that is offered. Moreover, the availability of the GSP option may have galvanized these men to a decision to improve, which decision was maintained even if the random allocation selected them to the usual services. In other words, the GSP may have represented a new hope to those who chose to be randomized, and not getting in to the GSP may not have extinguished this hope despite their being randomized to the control group.[6]

In conclusion, we suggest that future efforts to assist homeless substance abusers focus additional attention on issues of job readiness and employment, both opportunities and openings. This is the most difficult area to affect given the economic condition of our cities, but it is essential if these men are to restructure their time and lives away from cocaine and, hence, homelessness.

REFERENCES

1. Leaf PJ, Thompson KS, Lam JA, Jekel JF, et al. Partnerships in recovery: shelter-based services for homeless cocaine abusers: New Haven. Alcoholism Treatment Quarterly 1993; 10:77-90.

2. Fischer PJ. Alcohol, drug abuse and mental health problems among homeless persons: a review of the literature, 1980-1990. Rockville, Maryland: U.S. Dept. HHS, PHS, ADAMHA, March 1991, p. xxvii.

3. Spinner GF and Leaf PJ. Homelessness and drug abuse in New Haven. Hospital and Community Psychiatry 1992; 43:166-68.

4. Dean JA, Dean AG, Burton A, et al.. EPIINFO Version 5.0. Atlanta, GA: Centers for Disease Control, 1990.

5. McLellan AT, Luborsky L, Woody GE, O'Brien CP. Evaluation instrument for substance abuse patients: the Addiction Severity Index. Journal of Nervous and Mental Diseases 1980; 168:26-33.

6. Lam JA, Hartwell SW, Jekel JF. "I prayed real hard, so I know I'll get in.": Living with randomization. New Directions for Program Evaluation 1994; 63:55-66.

Homelessness and Substance Use Among Alcohol Abusers Following Participation in Project H&ART

Sandra C. Lapham, MD, MPH
Marge Hall, MA
Betty J. Skipper, PhD

SUMMARY. Project H&ART was a randomized intervention trial for homeless alcohol abusers in Albuquerque, N.M. Interventions were four months in duration and included: a high intensity program (case management plus peer-supervised housing), a medium intensity group (peer-supervised housing only); a housed, and a nonhoused control group. Clients were interviewed at baseline and re-interviewed ten months following program entry to determine substance use, housing stability and employment status. Program graduation rates were about 25% for the three housed groups. The outcome evaluation revealed significant within groups improvements in all of the outcomes,

Sandra C. Lapham, Marge Hall, and Betty J. Skipper are affiliated with The Lovelace Institutes, Institutes for Health and Population Research, 1650 University, NE, Suite 302, Albuquerque, NM 87102.

Address correspondence to Sandra C. Lapham, MD, MPH, Director, Substance Abuse Research Programs, The Lovelace Institutes, Lovelace Institute for Health and Population Research, 1650 University NE, Suite 302, Albuquerque, NM 87102.

This research was supported by Grant #5 U01 AA08815-02 from the National Institute on Alcohol Abuse and Alcoholism.

[Haworth co-indexing entry note]: "Homelessness and Substance Use Among Alcohol Abusers Following Participation in Project H&ART." Lapham, Sandra C., Marge Hall, and Betty J. Skipper. Co-published simultaneously in the *Journal of Addictive Diseases* (The Haworth Medical Press, an imprint of The Haworth Press, Inc.) Vol. 14, No. 4, 1995, pp. 41-55; and: *The Effectiveness of Social Interventions for Homeless Substance Abusers* (ed: Gerald J. Stahler) The Haworth Medical Press, an imprint of The Haworth Press, Inc., 1995, pp. 41-55. Single or multiple copies of this article are available from The Haworth Document Delivery Service [1-800-342-9678; 9:00 a.m. - 5:00 p.m. (EST)].

no between groups or racial outcome differences, and more favorable alcohol use and housing stability outcomes among program graduates than dropouts. On follow-up, women in the study had fewer days of alcohol use and had more days of stable housing, but were less likely to be employed, compared with men. We suggest that clients' personal motivation for recovery, rather than program-related factors, were most influential in determining outcomes. *[Article copies available from The Haworth Document Delivery Service: 1-800-342-9678.]*

INTRODUCTION

For decades research among homeless alcoholics consisted primarily of general descriptions of the sociodemographic characteristics of the population.[1] While descriptions of the population of interest are essential to an understanding of the problem, treatment solutions require information from scientific investigations regarding successful treatment strategies for this population.

Knowledge about the effectiveness of different interventions has been scarce.[2] However, as a result of the initiation of the Community Demonstration Program of the National Institute on Alcohol Abuse and Alcoholism, investigators began systematic studies of various treatment approaches,[2] and outcome studies are appearing more frequently in the literature.

The Lovelace Institutes, in collaboration with Health Care for the Homeless (HCH) and St. Martin's Hospitality Center (SMC), and with funding from the National Institute on Alcohol Abuse and Alcoholism, recently completed a prospective, randomized comparison of the efficacy of three intervention strategies for treating homeless persons with alcohol-related problems. The objectives of the Albuquerque project, entitled Project H&ART (Housing and Alcohol Research Team), were to determine: whether group assignment was associated with positive outcomes relating to substance use, residential stability, and employment; and whether individuals within the intervention groups, and among the race/ethnic and gender groups, improved differentially.

METHODS

Intervention Design

The study was conducted during the period October, 1990-December, 1993. The target population consisted of homeless, single adult alcohol abusers who had been in the Albuquerque area for at least three months. Clients were recruited into Project H&ART by staff of a day shelter for homeless persons, outreach or clinic staff of Albuquerque Health Care for the Homeless (HCH), or by one of the community agencies which provides other services to homeless persons.

Study participants were required to spend at least one night in a social model detoxification facility,[3] following which informed study participants received a baseline assessment before they were randomized into one of three intervention groups. The programs developed for Project H&ART are described in detail elsewhere.[4] Group 1, the high intensity group, received case management and substance abuse counselling services, along with four months of housing in four-plex apartment buildings staffed by residence managers who provided peer support. The medium intensity group, Group 2, received four months of housing in similar apartments with support services from peer residence managers. Clients in Group 2 were expected to seek treatment for their alcohol and drug abuse on their own initiatives, from services normally available in the community. The low intensity group, Group 3, received four months of apartment- or motel-based housing and no additional services.

In all three groups subjects were required to be abstinent from substances of abuse and were subjected to random, and "on demand" breath and urine testing. Those who could not maintain sobriety were discharged from the program. About halfway through the 16-month intervention phase, Group 3 housing services were discontinued due to safety concerns for staff and clients. Individuals randomized to the new low intensity nonhoused group (designated Group 4) received referrals and bus fare to local and statewide alcohol treatment agencies and were paid to provide health services utilization data at twice weekly check-ins. The only exception to the randomization process was that after two women were randomly assigned to the nonhoused control group a decision was made to randomize all subsequent female participants to one of the housed groups.

Measures

Baseline and follow-up testing included the following instruments: the Addiction Severity Index (ASI)[5] [modified for use by homeless individuals]; the Alcohol Dependence Scale (ADS);[6] and the Personal History Form (PHF).[7] Interviews were conducted at baseline (following completion of detoxification), and at ten months following the baseline interview (10-month follow-up). In addition to interviews, urine samples were collected at the 10-month follow-up and analyzed for substances of abuse (cocaine, amphetamines, sedatives, hallucinogens, or narcotics), and clients were breath tested for alcohol content using a breathalyzer. The ADS was administered at baseline and was used as the baseline indicator of the severity of alcohol-related problems.

Statistical Methods

Baseline characteristics of clients were examined and compared among race/ethnic, gender and intervention groups. We then examined program and study attrition. The baseline characteristics of those who stayed in the program were compared with those of program drop-outs, and drop-out rates were compared among the intervention and race/ethnic and gender groups. Study attrition was examined by comparing baseline characteristics of those who were interviewed at ten months and those who were lost to follow-up. We then examined changes in alcohol and drug use, and housing and employment patterns from baseline to follow-up. Outcomes were determined for all subjects at the 10-month follow-up. Statistical analyses were conducted only for those persons with known values for the variables under investigation. Those who had not used alcohol or drugs in the 30 days before the follow-up interview were classified into a "favorable" outcome status (Table 1). Employment stability was measured by responses to individual questions on the ASI and by ASI employment scale change scores. Housing stability was measured by responses to individual questions on the PHF. The Chi-square statistic was used in the analysis of contingency tables and the Kruskal-Wallis Test was used for comparing continuous variables.

General linear models were used to investigate differences in outcomes between intervention, race/ethnic, and gender groups. Multivariate models were developed for: days of alcohol use; days of stable housing, defined by the number of days not literally homeless or marginally housed (see Table 1) or in an institution; and days paid for employment in the 30 days before follow-up.

To control for problem severity at baseline, problem indicators (Table 1) were used as covariates in these models. A second set of models was created which included only members of Groups 1-3, to investigate whether time in the program (< 7 days; 7 or more days without graduating; graduated) was associated with favorable outcomes after controlling for other variables. These models were identical to the above models except that the ASI alcohol composite score was added (because univariate analyses revealed that ASI scores were associated with length of stay in the program).

TABLE 1. Favorable substance use outcome and baseline problem indicator definitions.

Substance Use Outcome Classification	Measure
Alcohol/Drug Use Outcome	
Favorable	No alcohol or drug use past 30 days
	Breathalyzer negative (if done)
	Drug screen negative (if done)
Medium	Number of days use to feel effects < 8 (past 30 days)
	No use of drugs except THC (past 30 days)
	Days experienced ARP = 0 (past 30 days)
	Days experienced DRP = 0 (past 30 days)
	Drug screen negative (except THC)
Problem Indicator	
Serious Alcohol Problem	ADS score = 22+
Drug Problem	Primary drug not alcohol OR ever injected any drug OR initial drug screen positive for any drug excluding marijuana
Housing Stability Problem	Total time homeless >2 years OR literal homeless 15+ days before admission
Employment Problem	Unemployed past year OR longest full time job <1 year
Legal Problem	Pending court action when entered Project H&ART OR trouble controlling violent behavior OR history of arrest for robbery, homicide, rape, assault
Medical Classification	ASI medical composite: 0; >0-.05; or >.05
Psychiatric Classification	ASI psychiatric composite: 0-.10; .11-.29; or .30+

ASI = Addiction Severity Index
THC = tetrahydrocannabinoids
ARP = Alcohol-related problems
DRP = Drug-related problems

Note: Literally homeless included: all-night theater, subway station, or other indoor public place; subway or bus; abandoned building; car or other private vehicle; on the street or in other outdoor place; and emergency shelter. Marginally housed included: hotel/motel; someone else's room, apartment, or house; and transitional housing. Institiutional homeless includes: hospital; nursing home; treatment or recovery program; jail or prison; or corrections halfway house.

RESULTS

Participation Rates and Client Baseline Characteristics

The program screened 980 persons, of whom 665 met the eligibility criteria, 497 entered the detoxification program, and 469 completed the detoxification program and were randomized to one of the intervention groups. Comparisons between characteristics of eligible clients who did and did not enter Project H&ART revealed that they were of similar age and had similar histories of alcohol-related problems and years of lifetime homelessness. One hundred sixty-one participants (34%) were randomized to Group 1; 164 (35%) to Group 2; 92 (20%) to Group 3; and 52 (11%) to the nonhoused control Group 4. Clients ranged in age from 18-67, with a median age of 37 years. Baseline comparisons among persons in the four intervention groups revealed no differences in age group, years of education, race/ethnicity, or classification as having alcohol, drug, housing stability, employment, or legal problems. In each of the groups over 85% of the clients reported alcohol as their primary substance of abuse.

The majority of the clients who entered Project H&ART were males; females represented only 13% of the client population. About 41% were non-Hispanic white (referred to subsequently as "white"); 31% Hispanic white (Hispanic); 18% Native American; and 10% belonged to other race groups. There were some differences in demographic characteristics among members of the different race/ethnic and gender groups. Whites had somewhat higher education levels, with about one third of the population having completed more than 12 years of school. Women were significantly less likely than men to be veterans.

Almost all of the clients (436/469, 93%) reported that alcohol was their drug of choice; 84% reported some alcohol use and 43% some drug use in the 30 days before program entry. Urine drug screens at baseline, collected at the time of discharge from the detoxification program, indicated that 14% of the clients had recently used a variety of substances other than alcohol. Baseline urine drug screens revealed that benzodiazepines (4%) and cannabinoids (4%) were the most commonly detected drugs, followed by barbiturates (3%) and amphetamines (2%). Over three quarters of the clients (78%) reported they had previously undergone treatment for alcohol-related problems. The ADS scores ranged from 0 to 46, with a mean of 22.5 (SD = 9.6) and a median of 23. A little over half of the clients had scores consistent with substantial or severe alcohol-related problems.

Native Americans and members of the "other race" group reported drinking for fewer years over their lifetimes compared to whites or Hispanics. Whites and Native Americans reported having been treated for alcohol abuse more times in the past than Hispanics or members of "other races"; and whites reported more days having experienced alcohol-related problems in the 30 days before admission, compared with "other races." However, mean ASI alcohol composite scores did not differ significantly among the race/ethnic groups. Native Americans reported significantly less drug use, and those belonging to the "other race" group reported more drug use, compared to whites and Hispanics. Women reported similar histories of alcohol-related problems, compared to men. However, they reported fewer days having experienced drug-related problems in the 30 days before program entry (0.6) compared to men (2.8) (p < .05).

The majority of clients (53%) reported that they had been homeless for at least one year prior to admission. The mean age at which clients reported first becoming homeless was 30.4 years. There were no significant race/ethnic differences in total years of homelessness, but women reported fewer total years homeless than men. Interview data concerning housing status in the 30 days before program entry revealed that clients, on average, spent 21 days housed, with no race/ethnic differences. Clients depended heavily on emergency shelters to meet their housing needs. About 50% spent at least one night in emergency shelters in the 30 nights prior to entering the detoxification facility. Only 7 persons (2%) had a stable housing situation at baseline and only 23% reported no literal homeless days in the 30 days before program admission. Women were less likely than men to have been literally homeless in the 30 days before program entry.

Almost half of the population identified their professions as skilled labor; an additional 25% were clerical workers, or semi- to unskilled laborers. The longest period of full-time employment averaged about four years, with Native Americans, those in the "other race" group, and females reporting fewer years, compared with Hispanic and white males. Approximately one quarter of the population had been employed full-time in the previous 12 months, and approximately half were unemployed in the previous 12 months before program admission. ASI employment composite scores were significantly higher among Hispanics and Native Americans, compared to whites and members of the "other race" group. Eighteen percent of the clients were classified at baseline as having an employment stability problem, with Native Americans and women more likely to be classified in this problem category.

More than one quarter of the population reported chronic medical problems. Forty-six percent of clients reported past histories of depression and 40% reported past histories of anxiety. There were no significant race/ethnic or gender differences in the ASI medical composite scores among clients, but women reported more psychiatric symptomatology, and whites reported more symptomatology than persons of other races.

Program and Study Attrition

On average, clients from Groups 1-3 stayed in the program for 67 days (median = 63 days) and about one quarter of the population graduated. There were no differences in retention rate by age group, race/ethnicity, or gender. Those with more than 12 years of education stayed in the program longer (mean = 73 days, SE = 3) than those with 12 years of education (71 days, SE = 3), or those with fewer than 12 years of education (55 days, SE = 4) (p < .01), but those with more than 12 years of education were not significantly more likely to graduate. Veterans stayed in housing longer than non-veterans, 64 days (SE = 3) versus 74 days (SE = 4) (p < .05). Persons who were classified as having a drug problem or legal problem had shorter mean lengths of stay in the program, compared with persons without these classifications.

There were no differences among the age, gender, marital status, education, or veteran status groups with respect to the reasons clients left the program. However, whites and persons of the "other race" group left more commonly for personal reasons (44% and 47%, respectively) compared to Hispanics (35%) and Native Americans (19%). Persons in the "other race" category left less commonly because of substance use (20%), compared to 43% for Hispanics, 44% for whites and 59% for Native Americans.

The overall follow-up rate for the 10-month interview was 78% (84% for females; 71% for white males; 86% for Hispanic males; 79% for Native American males; and 77% for other males. Hispanics had higher follow-up rates than the other groups (p < .05). There were no significant baseline differences in substance abuse, housing, or legal problem indicators between those who did and did not complete a follow-up interview. Persons classified as having an employment problem, however, were more likely to have received a 10-month follow-up interview than those who were not classified as having a problem.

A higher percentage of Group 1 clients (84%) received follow-up interviews, compared to members of the other groups; members of Group 2 had the lowest follow-up rates (75%) (p < .05). In addition, 88% of persons who graduated completed a follow-up interview, compared to 76% for those who did not graduate (χ^2 7.34, p <.01).

Comparisons Between Pre- and Post-Treatment Characteristics

One hundred three persons (32%) had no reported alcohol or drug use in the 30 days before the follow-up interview. About one quarter of the population had stable housing and one quarter were employed full-time (20 or more paid work days/30). Within groups comparisons revealed a significant decrease, from baseline to follow-up, in days of alcohol use, ASI alcohol composite scores, increased days of housing stability, increased number of days employed, and increased employment status in all of the intervention groups. There were no statistically significant within group differences in drug use between baseline and follow-up. Eighteen percent (54/308 of the follow-up drug screens) were positive for substances other than alcohol; 16% (51/329 of the breathalyzer tests at follow-up) were positive (> .02%). There were no between groups differences in breathalyzer or urine drug screen results.

There were 98 program graduates among the 331 persons in Groups 1-3 who received 10-month follow-up interviews. The graduates were more likely than nongraduates to have favorable substance use outcomes. Of the graduates, 54 persons (55%) had favorable outcomes and 13 persons (13%) had medium outcomes. In contrast, 46 nongraduates (20%) had favorable and 45 (20%) medium outcomes (Chi-square p <.001). The combined group of program graduates were somewhat more likely than nongraduates to be employed at the 10-month follow-up, with the differences approaching statistical significance. Thirty of the graduates (31%) were employed 20 or more days; 40 (41%) 1-19 days, and 27 (28%) were not employed. Among the nongraduates 46 (20%) were employed 20 or more days, 102 (44%) 1-19 days, and 85 (36%) were not employed (Chi-square p = .07).

Program graduates also were more likely to have stable housing than nongraduates. Thirty-nine (40%) of the graduates had stable housing for all 30 nights before the 10-month follow-up; 37 (38%) did not have stable housing for the entire period but had no nights of literal homelessness; and 21 (22%) had at least one night of literal homelessness. Among the nongraduates the corresponding figures were 35 (16%); 84 (39%); and 98 (45%) (Chi-square p < .001).

The multivariate models for the continuous outcome variables "days of alcohol use" and "days employed" were significant, statistically, but the model predicting the number of stable housing days was not (Table 2). Persons with more medical problems reported more days of alcohol use, and women reported significantly fewer days of alcohol use compared to men. As expected, longer intervals between the baseline and follow-up interviews were associated with more days of reported alcohol use.

The statistical models which included only persons in Groups 1-3 all reached statistical significance at the p < .001 level. These models revealed no associations between ASI alcohol composite scores and any of the

TABLE 2. Relationship among race, gender and favorable outcomes.

	Alcohol Use Days (past 30 days)		Stable Housing Days (past 30 days)		Employed Days (past 30 days)	
	Estimate (SE)	p-value	Estimate (SE)	p-value	Estimate (SE)	p-value
Age Regression Coefficient	−0.066 (.057)	NS	0.092 (.088)	NS	−0.181 (.057)	<.01
Baseline Severe Alcohol Problem						
No	5.2 (1.1)	NS	13.5 (1.7)	NS	8.1 (1.1)	NS
Yes	6.6 (1.1)		12.8 (1.6)		8.0 (1.1)	
Baseline Severe Drug Problem						
No	6.0 (1.1)	NS	13.4 (1.6)	NS	7.9 (1.1)	NS
Yes	5.8 (1.1)		12.8 (1.7)		8.2 (1.1)	
Baseline Employment Problem						
No	5.9 (1.1)	NS	13.6 (1.7)	NS	9.7 (1.1)	<.01
Yes	6.0 (1.1)		12.7 (1.7)		6.4 (1.1)	
Baseline Housing Stability Problem						
No	5.1 (1.0)	NS	16.1 (1.6)	<.001	10.0 (1.0)	<.001
Yes	6.8 (1.2)		10.2 (1.8)		6.2 (1.2)	
Baseline Legal Problem						
No	5.2 (1.1)	NS	13.7 (1.7)	NS	8.4 (1.1)	NS
Yes	6.6 (1.1)		12.6 (1.7)		7.7 (1.1)	

	Measure 1			Measure 2			Measure 3		
Baseline Medical Category									
0	4.3	(1.1)	<.05	13.6	(1.7)	NS	9.9	(1.1)	<.001
.01-.50	5.9	(1.3)		13.1	(1.9)		8.9	(1.3)	
.51+	7.6	(1.3)		12.7	(1.9)		5.4	(1.3)	
Baseline Psychiatric Category									
0-.105	5.4	(1.2)	NS	13.5	(1.8)	NS	7.4	(1.2)	NS
.106-.294	7.5	(1.2)		12.2	(1.8)		8.9	(1.2)	
.295+	4.9	(1.2)		13.7	(1.9)		7.8	(1.2)	
Race/Ethnicity									
White	6.5	(1.1)	NS	12.5	(1.7)	NS	8.7	(1.1)	NS
Hispanic	5.6	(1.5)		12.6	(1.7)		7.1	(1.1)	
Native American	8.1	(1.5)		11.6	(2.2)		6.2	(1.4)	
Other	3.5	(1.7)		15.8	(2.7)		10.2	(1.7)	
Gender									
Male	7.8	(0.8)	<.01	10.7	(1.3)	<.05	9.7	(0.8)	.05
Female	4.0	(1.5)		15.5	(2.3)		6.4	(1.5)	
Months Baseline to Follow-up									
5-10	3.3	(1.0)	<.01	14.0	(1.4)	NS	7.1	(0.9)	NS
11-15	7.1	(1.3)		12.7	(1.9)		7.0	(1.3)	
16+	7.4	(1.7)		12.7	(2.6)		10.2	(1.7)	
Group Assignment									
1	5.3	(1.1)	NS	13.9	(1.7)	NS	8.5	(1.1)	NS
2	7.4	(1.1)		11.0	(1.7)		7.8	(1.1)	
3	7.1	(1.3)		13.3	(2.0)		7.0	(1.3)	
4	3.8	(1.9)		14.4	(2.9)		8.8	(1.9)	
Overall Model	$F_{19,302} = 2.68$ <.001 $R^2 = .14$			$F_{19,303} = 1.52$ NS $R^2 = .09$			$F_{19,303} = 4.55$ <.001 $R^2 = .22$		

outcome variables. Female gender was associated with better alcohol use and housing stability outcomes but worse employment outcomes, compared with men, after controlling for the other variables (p < .05 for all three models): days of alcohol use (5.9, SE = 1.6 for females and 9.1, SE = 1.0 for males); days of stable housing (15.1, SE = 2.4 for females and 10.1, SE = 1.5 for males); and days employed (6.7, SE = 1.6 for females and 10.1, SE = 1.0 for males). Time in the program was associated with improved outcomes in all of the models. Days of alcohol use were 4.4 (SE = 1.3) for graduates; 8.1 (1.0) for those who stayed 7 or more days; and 10.1 (SE = 2.4) for those who stayed fewer than 7 days (p < .01). Days of stable housing were 17.7 (SE = 1.9) for graduates; 10.8 (SE = 1.5) for those who stayed 7 or more days; and 9.2 (SE = 3.5) for those who stayed fewer than 7 days (p < .001). Days employed were 9.9 (SE = 1.3) for graduates; 6.7 (SE = 1.0) for those who stayed 7 or more days; and 8.7 (SE = 2.3) for those who stayed fewer than 7 days (p < .05).

DISCUSSION

The project was intended to serve adult, homeless alcoholics living in Albuquerque. Analysis of the characteristics of clients enrolled in Project H&ART supported the conclusion that this demonstration program reached the population intended–almost all were primary alcohol abusers who had been homeless or were at risk of becoming homeless. The race/ethnic distribution of participants was similar to that anticipated, except that a higher proportion than expected were not members of the three race/ethnic groups under study. Also, fewer women than expected were enrolled.[3]

Outcome analyses indicated that there were significant within group improvements in alcohol use and employment status from baseline to 10-month follow-up for all the intervention groups. The improvement in alcohol use, and the absence of an association between group assignment and the outcomes tested, has several possible explanations. One explanation is that persons who enrolled in the program may have been motivated to change their patterns of abusive substance use and were able to accomplish this whether the intervention was minimal or extensive. All persons who enrolled in the study entered and completed the social model detoxification program, and persons in Groups 1-3 received a substantial level of services. These interactions with clients may have had a positive impact on their recovery from substance abuse. Another possible explanation is that the subjects may have entered the study at a time when they needed assistance most, at a low point. Perhaps they might have improved on their own without any assistance. Since all of the subjects received some services, it is not possible to determine the extent to which this may have occurred. It also is conceivable that clients may not actually have changed their substance use over the follow-up period. They may simply have overstated the extent of their alcohol abuse and other problems at the baseline interview to ensure that they received services. This possibility was minimized, however, by the study design, in which clients were already admitted to the program when the baseline interviews were conducted by research staff and clients were assured that their responses would not influence their group assignments nor program status. It has been observed that many people who seek treatment for substance abuse are more interested in taking a break from using, and are less interested in achieving long-term abstinence.[6] There is, therefore, some question as to whether clients were telling us what they thought we wanted to hear, or whether they were sincerely interested in changing their behaviors and situations.

The study had several limitations. First, the instruments used to measure changes in alcohol and drug use and employment were not designed for use in homeless populations and some clients had difficulties responding to all the questions. Also, the follow-up period was less than one year, and questions concentrated on a 30-day period before the interview. This period may not have represented a stable outcome condition. Second, the initiation of the randomized trial was concurrent with the establishment and implementation of the program. The intervention may have been evaluated too soon, before it had matured into a stable program. Inevitable periods of program variability may have resulted in reduced overall program effectiveness. If funding had been available to continue the project, it is possible that it would have been more successful in assisting clients to achieve stability and sobriety. Third, the duration of the intervention also may have been insufficient to enable clients to achieve residential stability. Perhaps if it were of longer duration there may have been more improvement in the case managed or the peer counseled groups. However, approximately 70% of the clients dropped out before the four months of housing ended, and this rate is fairly consistent among the three housed groups. Thus, the length of time of the program may not be the critical issue for achieving housing stability and sobriety. There may be other factors which also play a part in this process. It appears that certain clients were inherently motivated to change and others were not ready to make this change. Unfortunately, we have not been able to identify those who are ready to begin the process of recovery.

Finally, it became clear to staff that clients had different needs and desires at program entry. Some clients enrolled primarily because of the prospect of free housing. These persons had no interest in a recovery program. If assigned to Group 1 they left soon after it became apparent that they were in a structured program. Others really wanted to be in a structured, traditional treatment program and were assigned to the housed control group. This may have led to the high attrition rates demonstrated in all of the groups. A study in which clients had input into the group assignment decision may have yielded different results.

The statistical models did reveal some associations between baseline characteristics and outcome status. Persons with more medical problems (possibly related to their alcohol use) were less likely to have had favorable substance abuse outcomes and reported fewer days of employment prior to the follow-up interview. Favorable substance use outcomes were less likely if the client was classified as having a baseline drug or housing stability problem. Older age predicted more favorable substance abuse outcomes, but less favorable employment status. As expected, longer intervals between the baseline and follow-up interviews were associated with more days of reported alcohol use and less favorable substance use outcomes.

In conclusion, the program initiated for the present study experienced high attrition rates. The study retained its randomized design; one of the groups (the housed control group) was discontinued in the first year of operation and was replaced with a nonhoused control group. Comparisons of those who did and did not receive the 10-month follow-up interview revealed that the populations were similar in most respects. Outcome analysis revealed that on average clients in all of the intervention groups improved, with respect to their alcohol use and employment status. Race/ethnic outcome differences were minimal, but there were significant differences in improvement rates by gender. A higher percentage of women had favorable substance abuse outcomes, but women were less successful than men in gaining employment.

REFERENCES

1. Fischer PJ, and Breakey WR. The epidemiology of alcohol, drug, and mental disorders among homeless persons. American Psychologist, 1991, 46(11):1115-28.

2. Orwin RG, Goldman HH, Sonnefeld LJ, Ridgeley MS, Smith NG, Garrison-Mogren R, O'Neill E, and Sherman A. Alcohol and drug abuse treatment of homeless persons: results from the NIAAA community demonstration program. Journal of Health Care for the Poor and Underserved, 1994, 5(4):326-352.

3. Lapham SC, Hall M, Snyder J, Skipper BJ, McMurray-Avila M, Pulvino S, Kozeny T. Evaluation of a mixed social-medical model detoxification program for homeless alcoholics (Submitted).

4. Lapham SC, Hall M, McMurray-Avila M, Beaman H. Albuquerque's community-based housing and support services demonstration program for homeless alcohol abusers. Alcoholism Treatment Quarterly, 10(3-4), 1993.

5. McClellan AT, Luborsky L, Woody GE, & O'Brien CP. An improved diagnostic evaluation instrument for substance abuse patients. J. Neurons and Mental Disease, 1980, 168:26-33.

6. Skinner HA, and Horn JL. Alcohol Dependence Scale (ADS) user's guide. Addiction Research Foundation, Toronto, Canada, 1981.

7. Barrow SM, Hellman F, Lovell AM, Plapinger JD, Robinson CR, & Struening EL. Personal history follow-up. New York State Psychiatric Institute, New York, N.Y., 1985.

8. Rounsaville BJ, and Kleber HD. Psychotherapy/counseling for opiate addicts: Strategies for use in different treatment settings. Int J Addict. 1985, 20:869-896.

Eighteen-Month Follow-Up Data on a Treatment Program for Homeless Substance Abusing Mothers

Elizabeth M. Smith, PhD
Carol S. North, MD
Louis W. Fox, BS

SUMMARY. In response to the dearth of data on substance abuse treatment among homeless mothers, this study breaks new ground in presenting 18-month follow-up data on 149 homeless mothers with young children enlisted in a substance abuse treatment program. The effects of residential compared to nonresidential services were evaluated over the follow-up period. Although dropout rates were high, predictors of dropout were identified, and the residential had a lower dropout rate compared to the nonresidential comparison group. Members of both residential and nonresidential groups evidenced improvement in alcohol and drug problems and in housing stability, regardless of the amount of time they spent in the program. This project demonstrated that homeless mothers can be more successfully engaged in substance abuse programs with provisions of residential

Elizabeth M. Smith, Carol S. North, and Louis W. Fox are affiliated with the Department of Psychiatry, Washington University School of Medicine, St. Louis, MO.

Address correspondence to Elizabeth M. Smith, PhD, Washington University, School of Medicine, Department of Psychiatry, 4940 Children's Place, St. Louis, MO 63110.

This research was supported by National Institute on Alcohol Abuse and Alcoholism Grant #08804.

[Haworth co-indexing entry note]: "Eighteen-Month Follow-up Data on a Treatment Program for Homeless Substance Abusing Mothers." Smith, Elizabeth M., Carol S. North, and Louis W. Fox. Co-published simultaneously in the *Journal of Addictive Diseases* (The Haworth Medical Press, an imprint of The Haworth Press, Inc.) Vol. 14, No. 4, 1995, pp. 57-72; and: *The Effectiveness of Social Interventions for Homeless Substance Abusers* (ed: Gerald J. Stahler) The Haworth Medical Press, an imprint of The Haworth Press, Inc., 1995, pp. 57-72. Single or multiple copies of this article are available from The Haworth Document Delivery Service [1-800-342-9678; 9:00 a.m. - 5:00 p.m. (EST)].

57

placement in addition to participation in a therapeutic community. Future interventions can take advantage of this knowledge in designing more effective programs. *[Article copies available from The Haworth Document Delivery Service: 1-800-342-9678.]*

INTRODUCTION

In the general substance abuse literature, information on substance abuse in male populations far exceeds that in women. The special population of the homeless is no exception to this imbalance of knowledge. While some outcome data on substance abuse treatment for homeless men are starting to appear in the literature, virtually nothing is known about the effectiveness of substance abuse treatment programs for homeless women. Because treatment needs, programmatic considerations, and response to treatment among domiciled women are well known to differ from those of their male counterparts, one might anticipate important differences between homeless men and women regarding substance abuse treatment.

Given the dearth of data on substance abuse treatment among homeless mothers, this study breaks new ground in presenting treatment outcome data on a series of homeless mothers. This report provides information on baseline characteristics and 18-month follow-up treatment outcome data on 149 homeless mothers with young children who participated in a unique substance abuse program that tested the effects of residential compared to nonresidential services. The intervention was based on attaining recovery through a model of participants seeking sobriety helping each other in a modified therapeutic community setting with a 12-step program. The substance abuse program providing the source of data for this report was a joint venture between the Washington University School of Medicine and Grace Hill Neighborhood Services, integrating settlement house and recovery philosophies in one program. The project was funded by the National Institute on Alcohol Abuse and Alcoholism (NIAAA).

DESCRIPTION OF PROGRAM

The intervention design blended three approaches: (1) Grace Hill's settlement house philosophy of strengthening neighbors so that neighbors help one another; (2) traditional recovery services drawing on the 12-step approach in the context of group therapy; and (3) Yablonsky's theory of the therapeutic community in which addicts act as co-therapists.[1] The model that emerged was a modified therapeutic community, supported by professional recovery staff and programming, external 12-step groups, and Grace Hill neighbors and peers.

Previously or currently substance-abusing homeless mothers with young children were eligible for the program if they were homeless or in imminent danger of homelessness and they had one or more children ages 12 or younger in their care. A referral network was generated and cultivated for this program, and referral sources included the Grace Hill medical clinics, shelters and outreach programs for the homeless, substance abuse and mental health treatment programs in the community, local hospitals, existing neighborhood connections within the Grace Hill system and the community, word-of-mouth networks established by program staff, and activities such as open house events to increase community awareness. Before entering the program, subjects were randomly allocated to either the active intervention (i.e., seven mothers at a time living with their children at the Center) or to the control group (seven families making alternative living arrangements such as a shelter or with relatives but attending the day program at the center with their children). All women, regardless of housing assignment, participated in the same substance abuse treatment program.

In attempting to determine how most efficiently and economically the program goals could be met, this study compared the outcomes of women randomized to the residential group (i.e., those living at the Family Center) to those of women who attended only during the day and lived elsewhere during the first phase of the program. During this time, both groups received the same daily recovery and neighborhood services; the difference was that some were settled in the stable residence at the Center and others stayed in precarious, temporary living spaces.

The basic program, which lasted one year per family, offered two phases. Phase I was a 90-day module centered around a treatment/recovery model conducted in a substance-free, therapeutic community setting, with both group and individual treatment modalities. Upon graduation from Phase I, all families entered Phase II, where they lived in the community and continued to receive ongoing professionally facilitated support group participation and contact with the therapeutic community. A more detailed description of the program is provided in another publication.[2]

METHODS

Data Collection

Once a woman was determined to be eligible for the study, a baseline interview was conducted immediately prior to beginning the program. Follow-up assessments were scheduled at six, twelve, and eighteen months after baseline for a total of four assessment points. The assessment battery included the NIAAA core instruments (described in the introduction to this issue) along with several site-specific instruments. The Addiction Severity Index (ASI) (the primary source of substance abuse symptom level data) is a structured questionnaire administered by trained lay interviewers and assesses problem severity in seven areas commonly affected by alcohol and substance abuse: alcohol use, drug use, employment, medical status, legal status, social status, and psychiatric status. Higher scores on each composite indicate greater problem severity within that area. Like factor scores, the actual numeric value of any composite score has little intrinsic meaning and cannot be compared to other composite scores. Each score is used primarily to compare groups at each assessment and to quantify change across assessments.

A structured interview, the Diagnostic Interview Schedule (DIS)[3] was administered at baseline. The DIS was used to make DSM-III-R diagnoses, including major depression, panic disorder, generalized anxiety disorder, post-traumatic stress disorder, alcohol abuse or dependence, drug abuse or dependence, and antisocial personality disorder. A supplement to the Personal History Form (PHF) was developed at the St. Louis project site to gather more detailed information on subjects' pattern of housing.

Data Analysis

Baseline sociodemographic characteristics and candidate predictor variables were examined using descriptive statistics, bivariate statistical tests (t-tests for numerical measures and chi-square tests for categorical measures), and bivariate plots.

A study subject was classified as a "no-show" if she was accepted into the program, completed the baseline assessment, and then did not begin the program. Analyses of the predictors of being a no-show were conducted using contingency tables, univariate logistic regression, and hierarchical multivariate logistic regression models.[4]

Dropout from the program was defined as leaving the program prior to successful completion for any reason for participants who actually began the program. Estimates of the rate of dropout were made using the product-limit method of survival analysis[5-7] and multivariate Cox proportional hazard models.[6,7] For these analyses, participants who had successfully completed the program were censored at the time they graduated from the program, and those who were still in the program at the end of the study were censored at the time the program was terminated.

Candidate predictors for the analyses of no-shows and dropouts in-

cluded treatment group assignment; baseline sociodemographic characteristics; history of previous alcohol or drug treatment; patterns of alcohol
abuse, drug abuse, and homelessness; and measures of employment and
socialization and psychiatric diagnoses assessed from the DIS. Also included in the analysis of dropouts was the amount of time spent in Phase I
and whether the participant completed Phase I.

Longitudinal outcomes were examined using a set of longitudinal data
analytic techniques known as mixed models.[8-12] The following outcomes
were examined: alcohol use composite score, drug use composite score,
employment composite score, and housing stability score. The alcohol and
drug use composite scores measured severity of alcohol use and their impact on the subject's recent life. The employment composite score was a
measure of the level of employment and the severity of the subject's employment problems. The housing stability score was an adjusted measure
for the percentage of time the subject spent in stable housing during the
time between each assessment, and it quantified the permanence and independence of the subject's housing. This score was derived from the PHF
Supplement. Adjustments included number of moves made during the
period, types of all housing attained, level of independence, and reasons
why the subject moved away from each housing situation. A similar housing stability score was calculated from the PHF administered at the baseline assessment covering the 60-day period prior to the interview. The
housing stability score ranged from zero to one, with higher scores indicating greater housing permanence and independence.

Candidate predictors for the analyses of longitudinal outcome included:
treatment group assignment; baseline sociodemographic characteristics; history of previous alcohol or drug treatment; patterns of alcohol abuse, drug
abuse, and homelessness; measures of employment and socialization; and
comorbid psychiatric diagnoses. Also included in the models were the
following measures: participation in any alcohol or drug abuse treatment
after leaving the Grace Hill program, types of alcohol and drug abuse treatment subjects received, length of stay in Phase I, length of stay in the overall
program, whether the subject successfully completed Phase I, whether the
subject successfully completed the program, and composite scores derived
from the ASI.

RESULTS

Participant Flow and Baseline Characteristics

A total of 149 women accepted into the program were included in the
analyses. Sixty-seven (45%) were assigned to the residential treatment

group and 82 (55%) were assigned to the nonresidential treatment group. (More women received random assignment to the nonresidential group because there was greater dropout and thus turnover in this group, which left more slots available for inclusion in the randomization pool.) Twenty-three women (15%) never began the Grace Hill program (i.e., were no-shows), 17 from the nonresidential group and 6 from the residential group. Of the 126 women who began the program, 107 (85%) left prior to completion (i.e., were dropouts), 10 (8%) completed the program, and 9 (7%) were still in the program at the time the program ended. Overall follow-up over the 18-month period was 90%.

Table 1 shows the demographic characteristics and lifetime psychiatric diagnoses of the groups. On average, the women were about 30 years of age, and virtually all were African-American. The majority had never married, and very few were currently married. They averaged three to four children apiece, with approximately three dependent children. Almost none of the women were working. With the exception of antisocial personality disorder, no statistically significant differences were found in any of the demographic variables between the residential and nonresidential groups. The women in the nonresidential group had a 3.3 times higher rate of antisocial personality disorder than the women in the residential group.

The women's baseline patterns of alcohol use, drug use, and homelessness are presented in Table 2. The relatively low number of days drinking and a relatively low alcohol use composite score (.20 ± .25) indicate that alcohol use, although a problem in these women, was not their major source of difficulty. Nonresidential women reported significantly more years of drinking to intoxication than did women in the residential group. The drug of choice was clearly cocaine, although the women averaged more years of experience with cannabis. Half (52%) of the women had been homeless more than once. The most frequent etiologic factor to which they ascribed their homelessness was economic problems, followed by substance abuse problems, and interpersonal conflict.

Never Began Program

Results of the final logistic regression model of no-shows are presented in Table 3. The model consisted of six variables: treatment group assignment, drug use composite score, ever-married marital status, amount of money received from public assistance in the past month, alcohol and drug problems reported as a reason for the current episode of homelessness, and other miscellaneous problems the women identified as reasons for their current episode of homelessness. There were no statistically significant interactions between any of the variables.

TABLE 1. Baseline sociodemographic characteristics and prevalence of psychiatric disorders of Grace Hill women by treatment group.

	Residential (N = 67)	Nonresidential (N = 82)	Total (N =149)
Age (years)	29.4 ± 4.8	30.1 ± 5.3	29.8 ± 5.1
Ethnic Background			
African-American	98.5%	96.3%	97.3%
White or other	1.5%	3.7%	2.7%
Marital Status			
Married	0.0%	2.4%	1.3%
Widowed	0.0%	3.7%	2.1%
Divorced	9.0%	8.5%	8.7%
Separated	28.4%	19.5%	23.5%
Single	62.7%	65.9%	64.4%
Number of Children	3.9 ± 1.6	3.5 ± 1.6	3.7 ± 1.6
Number of Dependents	3.2 ± 1.6	2.9 ± 1.6	3.0 ± 1.6
Education (years)[a]	11.3 ± 1.7	11.3 ± 1.3	11.3 ± 1.5
Employment			
Working	4.5%	2.4%	3.4%
Looking for work	41.8%	46.3%	44.3%
Not looking for work	46.3%	46.3%	46.3%
Disabled	3.0%	2.4%	2.7%
Other	4.5%	2.4%	3.4%
	(N = 66)	(N = 76)	
Psychiatric Disorder[b]			
Alcohol Use Disorder	45.5%	45.1%	47.2%
Substance Use Disorder			
Cannabis	16.7%	17.1%	16.9%
Cocaine	84.8%	81.6%	83.1%
Major Depression	7.6%	14.5%	11.3%
Antisocial Personality[c]	9.1%	25.0%	17.6%
Post-Traumatic Stress Disorder	22.7%	22.4%	22.5%
Panic Disorder	1.5%	2.6%	2.1%
Generalized Anxiety Disorder	6.1%	5.3%	5.6%

[a] Where GED = 12 years
[b] N = 7 women did not complete a DIS interview.
[c] $p < 0.05$

TABLE 2. Patterns of alcohol abuse, drug abuse, and homelessness in Grace Hill women by treatment group.

	Residential (N = 67)	Nonresidential (N = 82)	Total (N =149)
Alcohol Use			
Past month (days)	7.2 ± 9.6	8.1 ± 9.5	7.7 ± 9.5
Lifetime (years)	3.8 ± 5.5	5.4 ± 6.4	4.7 ± 6.0
Drinking to Intoxication			
Past month (days)	6.0 ± 9.1	6.9 ± 8.9	6.5 ± 9.0
Lifetime (years)[a]	3.1 ± 4.8	4.9 ± 6.0	4.1 ± 5.6
Cannabis Use			
Past month (days)	1.9 ± 5.5	1.8 ± 3.9	1.8 ± 4.7
Lifetime (years)	4.5 ± 5.1	5.4 ± 4.9	5.0 ± 5.0
Cocaine/Crack Use			
Past month (days)	11.0 ± 10.5	12.9 ± 11.5	12.0 ± 11.0
Lifetime (years)	3.1 ± 2.1	3.9 ± 3.2	3.5 ± 2.8
Any Drug Use			
Past month (days)	12.2 ± 11.1	14.0 ± 11.6	13.2 ± 11.4
Lifetime (years)[b]	7.3 ± 5.4	8.7 ± 5.6	8.1 ± 5.5
Age First Problematic Cannabis Use[c]	17.5 ± 4.6	17.6 ± 4.1	17.6 ± 4.4
Age First Problematic Cocaine Use[c]	25.9 ± 4.9	26.3 ± 6.0	26.1 ± 5.5
Age First Homeless	25.2 ± 6.3	25.4 ± 7.9	25.3 ± 7.2
Reasons Now Homeless			
Economic	67.2%	67.1%	67.1%
Drug/Alcohol related	52.2%	58.0%	56.4%
Interpersonal conflict	34.3%	31.7%	32.9%
Health related	3.0%	7.3%	5.4%
Safety concerns	25.4%	29.3%	27.5%
Other	22.4%	18.3%	20.1%

[a] $p < 0.05$
[b] $p < 0.10$
[c] estimated from DIS

Adjusting for the other variables in the model, subjects in the nonresidential treatment group were 3.2 times more likely to be no-shows than were subjects in the residential treatment group. The risk of being a no-show was increased for subjects who had ever married, who reported alcohol and drug problems as a reason for current homelessness, and who reported other miscellaneous problems as a reason for current homelessness. The risk of being a no-show was lower for subjects with greater severity of substance abuse at baseline, as measured by the drug use composite score, and for subjects receiving greater amounts of money from public assistance.

TABLE 3. Results of final models for never beginning Grace Hill program and for the rate of dropout from the Grace Hill program.

	Risk Ratio[a]	95% CI[b]	Chi-square	P
Never Began Program (Logistic)				
Nonresidential Assignment	3.23	1.05-9.95	4.19	0.04
Drug-Use Composite Score (at mean of 0.2)	0.30	0.11-0.82	5.59	0.02
Money from Public Assistance (at mean of $320)	0.15	0.04-0.62	6.88	0.01
Alcohol/Drug Problems Caused Homelessness	4.45	1.23-16.1	5.18	0.02
Other Problems Caused Homelessness	7.20	1.53-34.5	6.22	0.01
Ever Been Married	3.23	1.12-9.33	4.71	0.03
Rate of Dropout from Program (Cox)				
Nonresidential Assignment	1.83	1.19-2.82	7.58	0.01
Antisocial Personality	2.21	1.24-3.95	7.27	0.01
Number of Close Friends (at mean of 1 friend)	0.86	0.74-1.01	3.29	0.07
Alcohol to Intoxication (at mean of 4 years)	1.17	1.01-1.35	4.34	0.04
Live with Drug User	0.58	0.36-0.94	4.94	0.03
Weeks in Phase I (at 8 weeks)	0.51	0.26-1.00	3.83	0.05

[a] For the logistic regression model, the risk ratio is the odds ratio. For the Cox models, the risk ratio is the hazard ratio.

[b] 95% CI is the 95% confidence interval for estimated risk ratio.

Dropout from Program

Figure 1 shows the rate of dropout from the Grace Hill program for those women who actually began the program ($N = 126$) by treatment group assignment. Approximately 50% of the nonresidential group had left the pro-

FIGURE 1. Rate of Dropout for Grace Hill women who began by treatment group.

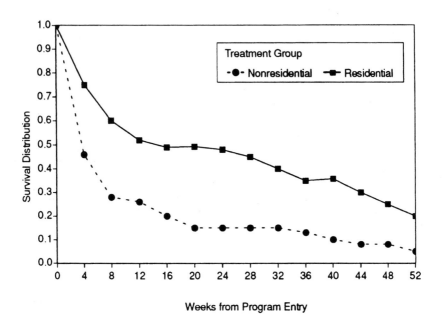

Weeks from Program Entry

gram by the fourth week compared to only about 25% of the residential group. At the twelve week mark (the planned length of Phase I), more than 75% of the nonresidential group had left the program compared to approximately 50% of the residential group.

Table 3 shows the results of the final Cox model of the rate of dropout. The model consisted of six variables: treatment group assignment, DIS diagnosis of antisocial personality disorder, number of close friends, number of years of drinking to intoxication, living with a drug user, and number of weeks spent in Phase I. There were no statistically significant interactions between any of the variables.

Adjusting for the other variables in the model, the rate of dropout was 1.8 times greater for participants assigned to the nonresidential treatment group compared to participants assigned to the residential treatment group. The rate of dropout was also increased for subjects who had a DIS diagnosis of antisocial personality disorder and for subjects with longer lifetime histories of drinking to intoxication. There was a protective effect (i.e., the rate of dropout was reduced) for subjects who reported having one or more close friends, who lived with a drug user (although this could also include shelter mates), and who spent more time in Phase I.

Longitudinal Outcome

The final model of predictors of the change in the alcohol use composite score over time included the following variables: treatment group assignment, interaction between treatment group assignment and time (as represented by the assessment point), lifetime history of drinking to intoxication, any previous treatment for alcohol abuse, attendance in a 12-step program after leaving the Grace Hill program, drug use composite score, and psychiatric composite score. Change in the alcohol use composite score over time by treatment group adjusted for the other variables included in the model is shown in Figure 2A. Adjusting for the other variables in the model, the overall alcohol use composite score did not differ between the residential and nonresidential treatment groups at any of the assessment points nor did it differ within treatment groups between any of the assessment points.

Greater lifetime history of drinking to intoxication and prior treatment for alcohol abuse were associated with higher mean alcohol use composite

FIGURE 2A. Alcohol-Use Composite Score by Treatment Group.

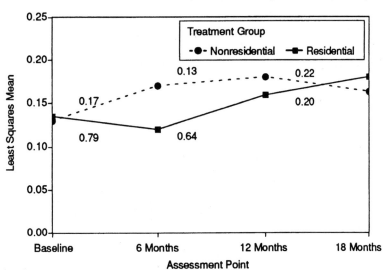

Note: p-value of change from baseline is beside line

scores during the study. Participation in a 12-step program on completion of the program was associated with lower alcohol use scores. Severity of alcohol use composite score was associated with drug use and psychiatric composite scores over time.

The final model of the drug use composite score over time included the following variables: treatment group assignment, interaction of treatment group assignment and time (as represented by the assessment point), number of years of drug use, alcohol use composite score, psychiatric composite score, and portion of time spent in literal or marginal homelessness in the past 60 days. Change in the drug use composite score over time by treatment group assignment adjusted for the other variables in the model is shown in Figure 2B. Adjusting for the other variables in the model, the overall drug use composite score did not differ between the residential and nonresidential treatment groups at any of the assessment points. Drug use composite scores did decrease significantly over time in both treatment groups. The drug use composite score over time was associated with greater lifetime history of drug use, severity of alcohol use and psychiatric composite scores over time, and portion of time spent in literal or marginal homelessness in the past 60 days at each assessment point.

The final model of the housing stability score over time contained the

FIGURE 2B. Drug-Use Score by Treatment Group.

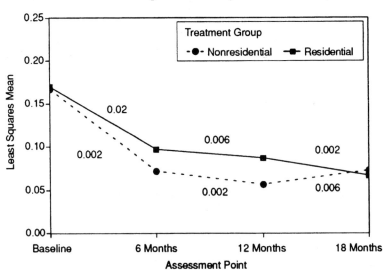

Note: p-value of change from baseline is beside line

following variables: treatment group assignment, interaction between treatment group and time (as represented by the assessment point), participation in alcohol or drug treatment after leaving the Grace Hill program, psychiatric composite score, and legal status composite score. Change in the housing stability score over time by treatment group adjusted for the other variables included in the model is shown in Figure 2C. Adjusting for the other variables in the model, the overall housing stability score did not differ between the residential treatment group and the nonresidential treatment group at any assessment point. Both treatment groups showed significant improvements in housing stability over time. Predictors of lower overall housing stability scores were more severe psychiatric or legal composite scores, and participation in substance abuse treatment after leaving the Grace Hill program.

The final model of the employment composite score over time consisted of the following variables: treatment group assignment, interaction between treatment group and time (as represented by the assessment point), amount of time the subject was in the program, and previous treatment for alcohol or drug abuse. Change in the employment composite score over time by treatment group adjusted for the other variables included in the model is shown in Figure 2D. Adjusting for the other vari-

FIGURE 2C. Housing Stability Score by Treatment Group.

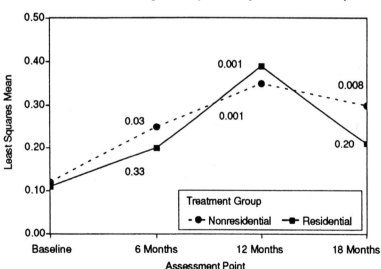

Note: p-value of change from baseline is beside line

FIGURE 2D. Employment Composite Score by Treatment Group.

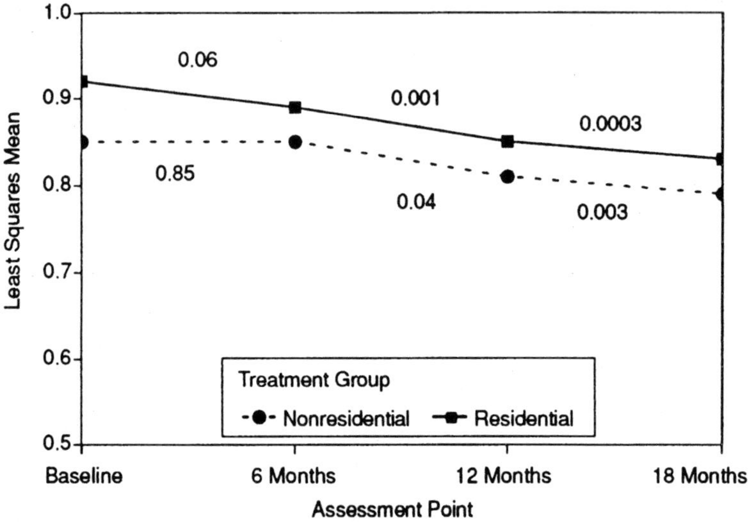

Note: p-value of change from baseline is beside line

ables in the model, there was no difference in the overall employment composite score between the residential and nonresidential treatment groups at any assessment point. Both treatment groups, however, showed significant improvement in employment, although the employment composite score was still, on average, in the very extreme severity range. Higher (more severe) employment composite scores over time were significantly associated with lack of prior substance abuse treatment and with greater amount of time spent in the Grace Hill program.

DISCUSSION

The most salient findings of this study were the low participation and retention rates: a 15% no-show rate and, among participants who actually started the program, an 85% dropout rate. Dismal as these rates might seem, however, significant predictors of no-shows and dropouts were found in the present study that might help guide future interventions. The rates from this study are compared to those of other studies that found dropout rates of 75%[13] and greater than 80%[14] for alcohol treatment programs over periods of 3-4 months, 68% for a substance abuse treatment program over 6 months,[15] and 58%-90% in a drug treatment program over 6-9 months.[16] Therefore the dropout rate in this study, while very discouraging, is not so remarkable. Difficulties in subject retention and limited success of substance abuse programs are well documented also in non-homeless populations. These difficulties are expected to be compounded in homeless populations, where experience has encountered serious complications in treatment of other psychiatric and other medical conditions. The data from the present study suggest poor effectiveness and low cost effectiveness of the present model of substance abuse treatment for this population.

A positive finding of the investigation was that women in all groups improved especially in drug use and housing stability regardless of the amount of time spent in the program. A possible explanation for this is that the mere admission of one's substance abuse problem and actively seeking help for it may represent a turning point for these women that resolves them toward recovery regardless of formal interventions. Another possibility is that even modest exposure to treatment significantly improves the woman's functioning and reduces drug use.

Potentially the most useful finding of the study was that subjects assigned to the residential group had lower rates of program dropout. Therefore, it appears that homeless women can be more successfully engaged in substance abuse treatment programs through their need for housing. Although other variables related to alcohol and drug abuse outcome and housing and employment stability did not seem to be affected by assignment group in the long term, the mere fact of higher retention in the residential group suggests possibilities for better results with more attention to programmatic features among those who do remain engaged. By combining the improved subject retention achieved by attention to residential needs with innovative programmatic efforts, additional gains in substance abuse treatment outcome for homeless families might be forthcoming.

REFERENCES

1. Yablonsky L. The Therapeutic Community: A Successful Approach for Treating Substance Abusers. New York: Gardner Press, 1989.

2. Smith EM, North CS, Heaton TM. A substance abuse recovery program for homeless mothers with children: St. Louis. Alcoholism Treatment Quarterly, 1993; 10(3/4):91-100.

3. Robins LN, Helzer JE, Cottler L, Golding E. NIMH Diagnostic Interview Schedule, Version III Revised. St. Louis, MO: Washington University, 1989.

4. Hosmer DW, Lemeshow S. Applied Logistic Regression. New York: John Wiley & Sons, 1989.

5. Kaplan EL, Meier P. Nonparametric estimation from incomplete observations. JASA, 1958; 53:457-481.

6. Kalbfleisch JD, Prentice RL. The Statistical Analysis of Failure Time Data. New York: John Wiley and Sons, 1980.

7. Cox DR, Oakes D. Analysis of Survival Data. London: Chapman and Hall, 1984.

8. Laird NM, Ware JH. Random-effects models for longitudinal data. Biometrics, 1982; 38:963-974.

9. Jennrich RI, Schluchter MD. Unbalanced repeated-measures models with structured covariance matrices. Biometrics, 1986; 42:805-820.

10. Schluchter MD. Analysis of incomplete multivariate data using linear models with structured covariance matrices. Stat Med, 1994.

11. Gibbons RD, Hedeker MA, Waternaux C, Davis JM. Random regression models: A comprehensive approach to the analysis of longitudinal psychiatric data. Psychopharmacol Bull, 1988; 24:438-443.

12. Vacek PM, Mickey RM, Bell DY. Application of two-stage random effects model to longitudinal pulmonary function data from sarcoidosis patients. Stat Med, 1989; 8:189-200.

13. Lapham SC, Hall M, Murray-Avila M, Beaman H. Albuquerque's community-based housing and support services demonstration program for homeless alcohol abusers. Alcoholism Treatment Quarterly, 1993; 10:139-154.

14. Stark MJ. Dropping out of substance abuse treatment: A clinically oriented review. Clin Psychol Rev, 1992; 12:93-116.

15. Pope AR, Conrad KJ, Baxter W, Elbaum P, Lisiecki MA, Daghestani A, Hultman C, Lyons J. Case managed residential care for homeless addicted veterans: Evanston/VA. Alcoholism Treatment Quarterly, 1993; 10:155-169.

16. Stahler GJ, Shipley TE, Bartelt D, Westcott D, Griffith E, Shandler I. Retention issues in treating homeless polydrug users: Philadelphia. Alcoholism Treatment Quarterly, 1993; 10:201-215.

Treatment Outcome as a Function of Treatment Attendance with Homeless Persons Abusing Cocaine

Joseph E. Schumacher, PhD
Jesse B. Milby, PhD
Ellen Caldwell, MS
James Raczynski, PhD
Molly Engle, PhD
Max Michael, MD
James Carr

SUMMARY. This research examines the influence of treatment attendance at two substance abuse outpatient treatment programs of the Birmingham Substance Abuse Homeless Project on substance abuse, homelessness, and unemployment outcomes with homeless persons abusing primarily crack cocaine. Results revealed that significant reductions across a one year period in alcohol use, cocaine use, and

Joseph E. Schumacher, Jesse B. Milby, Ellen Caldwell, James Raczynski, and Molly Engle are affiliated with The University of Alabama at Birmingham School of Medicine, Division of Preventive Medicine, Behavioral Medicine Unit.

Max Michael and James Carr are affiliated with the Birmingham Health Care for Homeless Coalition.

Address correspondence to Joseph E. Schumacher, PhD, The University of Alabama at Birmingham, 1717 11th Avenue South, 401 Medical Towers, Birmingham, AL 35205.

This research was supported by grant AA08819-01 from the National Institute on Alcoholism and Alcohol Abuse and National Institute on Drug Abuse.

[Haworth co-indexing entry note]: "Treatment Outcome as a Function of Treatment Attendance with Homeless Persons Abusing Cocaine." Schumacher, Joseph E. et al. Co-published simultaneously in the *Journal of Addictive Diseases* (The Haworth Medical Press, an imprint of The Haworth Press, Inc.) Vol. 14, No. 4, 1995, pp. 73-85; and: *The Effectiveness of Social Interventions for Homeless Substance Abusers* (ed: Gerald J. Stahler) The Haworth Medical Press, an imprint of The Haworth Press, Inc., 1995, pp. 73-85. Single or multiple copies of this article are available from The Haworth Document Delivery Service [1-800-342-9678; 9:00 a.m. - 5:00 p.m. (EST)].

73

homelessness were more likely to occur in clients who attended an average of 4.1 treatment days per week (High attendance or Enhanced Care group) than clients who attended less than one day a week on the average (Low attendance or Usual Care and Medium attendance groups). These results are consistent with the literature suggesting that more intensive contact early in treatment results in better long-term outcome with cocaine abusers, but has now been demonstrated with homeless cocaine abusers who have additional problems associated with housing and employment. *[Article copies available from The Haworth Document Delivery Service: 1-800-342-9678.]*

A continuity of care exists in the treatment of alcohol and drug abuse problems, ranging from brief interventions to more intensive and long-term treatment regimes. The usefulness of brief interventions generally has been established for persons with low levels of alcohol dependence.[1] For cocaine abuse, however, low attendance in psychotherapy has been found to be insufficient to produce remission in most patients and has been associated with difficulties in retaining clients in treatment.[2] Due to mood distress, depression and heightened craving associated with abstinence among cocaine abusers during the early stages of treatment, any form of treatment based on a once-a-week model is likely to be ineffective.[3]

A number of studies of drug abuse treatment effectiveness has related positive outcomes with time spent during treatment and length of time in treatment. Longer stays in treatment have been found to result in greater decreases in drug use, criminal activity, and unemployment.[4-7] For example, in the Treatment Outcome Prospective Study (TOPS), time spent in treatment (6 to 12 months) was among the most important predictors of post-treatment drug abuse for all types of drugs, except for cocaine.[5] The authors attributed this exception more to the growth in cocaine abuse during the time of the study than to the characteristics of the treatment.

Comprehensive, intensive, and multifaceted outpatient programs have been found to be the most successful at treating cocaine and crack cocaine addictions.[8,9] Such programs have included psychoeducation, urine testing, individual counseling, family counseling, group counseling, and relapse prevention. Intensive treatment requires clients to participate at a level that involves contacts several times per week with the treatment program.[10] Washton and his colleagues studied treatment outcome data of 63 chronic cocaine abusers who participated in six months of intensive outpatient treatment.[9] They reported that success rates were directly related to length of time in treatment, that is, longer time in treatment was related to more successful abstinence. Crucial elements of their outpatient rehabilitation program for crack cocaine abusers included an initial two-month, three days per week, intensive component plus a six-month relapse-prevention program. An eighty percent treatment completion rate and decreased referrals to inpatient care were found. Intensive, almost daily contact with the program in the early stages of abstinence was believed to be critical to the success of substance abuse treatment with cocaine abusers.[11-13]

Effective retention and treatment of cocaine abusers who are also homeless has only recently been demonstrated. A model outpatient day treatment program providing multiple contacts per week was effective with cocaine abusers, but was unsuccessful in treating homeless cocaine abusers with a 100% dropout rate before completing treatment.[14] Higgins and his colleagues were successful in treating cocaine abusers with less frequent contact in a behavioral reinforcement intervention, but none of their clients were homeless.[15] The Birmingham Substance Abuse Homeless Project developed an intensive two-month day treatment program followed by a drug-free work therapy and housing component (Enhanced Care) targeted at homeless cocaine abusers. The Enhanced Care program was successful in retaining clients and reducing alcohol and cocaine use and homelessness over a 12-month period in intensive day treatment as compared to a less intensive usual care program (Usual Care).[16,17]

The purpose of this report is to discuss how treatment attendance during the first two months of outpatient substance abuse treatment of Birmingham Substance Abuse Homeless Project affected treatment outcome in the areas of substance abuse, homelessness, and employment with cocaine abusers who were also homeless. After demonstrating the efficacy of the Enhanced Care intervention as compared to the Usual Care intervention on three of four major outcome variables (alcohol use, cocaine use, and homelessness) as reported elsewhere,[17] further investigation into the impact of the degree of treatment participation or attendance for all clients during the initial outpatient component of the project was conducted. It was hypothesized that more intense contact with the treatment program during the first two months of outpatient treatment would improve long-term outcome in cocaine abusers who were also homeless.

METHODOLOGY

Subjects

Volunteer participants were identified and screened for homelessness and substance abuse by project staff at the Birmingham Health Care for the Homeless Coalition (BHCHC). Substance dependency was based on DSM III-R criteria[18] and criteria for homelessness were derived from the 1987 Stuart B. McKinney Homeless Assistance Act, Public Law 100-77. Descriptions of the client sample are presented later.

Procedure

A randomized, two-group, controlled-comparison design with repeated measures was utilized for comparison of an enhanced day treatment program versus usual care. A total of 176 homeless persons with substance use disorders provided informed consent and were randomly assigned to one of two treatment groups: Enhanced Care and Usual Care. A standardized outcome battery[16] assessing alcohol use, other drug use (EMIT urine toxicologies), homelessness, and unemployment was administered by research interviewers who were blind to each subject's group assignment at four time points: baseline, 2-months, 6-months, and 12-months.

Usual Care consisted of twice weekly individual and group counseling, medical evaluation and treatment and/or referral for identified medical conditions. Referrals for housing and vocational services were made to other agencies, with the counselors serving as case managers. Education about AIDS and a monthly social support activity called "Club Birmingham" was also available to the Usual Care clients.

Enhanced Care was based on a state-of-the-art day treatment model where weekday attendance was expected for two months. The day treatment included a "therapeutic community," a patient self-government meeting in which patients reviewed contract goals and provided support and encouragement. Group therapy was scheduled three times per week. Multiple psychoeducational groups on various topics were also offered, such as, relapse prevention, social skills training, goal review, week-end planning, community resources for the homeless, etc. Individual counseling was scheduled weekly. Each client had individually-determined, objectively-defined goals to address major problems identified at initial assessment that were reviewed and modified weekly. After two months of day treatment and at least two weeks of abstinence, subjects graduated to a four-month work therapy and drug-free housing program which is discussed in greater detail elsewhere.[16,17]

Statistical Analysis

For purposes of analysis of the effect of treatment attendance on treatment outcome, all subjects from both treatment groups were combined and categorized into three treatment attendance groups (Low, Medium, and High) based on the following rationale and procedure. The Low attendance group was designated to capture those clients who were still ambivalent about seeking treatment and dropped out early or who intentionally entered the study only to claim the $15 baseline assessment fee. The Medium attendance group was designated to characterize typical attendance by clients seeking substance abuse services at BHCHC before the inception of the project. Finally, the High attendance group was designated to represent a level of participation expected by clients attending a more intensive outpatient program. The number of treatment days per week during the two-month outpatient component of treatment were rank ordered for all subjects and three attendance groups were identified based on logical cut points. These cut points and measures of central tendency are presented in the results section below.

This study's longitudinal design allows examination of individual's changing responses over time and comparison of treatment effectiveness at three levels of program attendance. Statistical methods must account for the dependence among successive observations made on each subject and handle incomplete data from individual subjects. The parametric assumptions underlying classical longitudinal methods such as repeated measures MANOVA and ANOVA were not met for the outcome measures studied. At each time point the outcome measures were extremely non-normal and there were many missing values at each follow-up point. Consequently, a nonparametric test proposed by Wei-Lachin was used.[19,20] The Wei-Lachin test is appropriate for both incomplete ordinal data and highly non-normal continuous data. At each time point a test statistic of medians is computed to compare groups; a linear combination of these statistics is formed for a multivariate omnibus test of group differences across all time points. Wei-Lachin test were calculated using a Fortran program created by Charles Davis.[21]

RESULTS

Subjects

Of the 176 clients who entered the study, 131 (74%) were exposed to some treatment and completed at least one follow-up interview. The follow-up rate for all subjects across all time points (2-, 6-, and 12-months) was 67.9%. There was no significant difference in attrition across follow-up time points. This sample was primarily male (79.4%), African-American (96.2%), high school-educated (mean years education 12.2, $SD = 2.1$), and crack cocaine-abusing (71.8%) with an average age of 35.8 ($SD = 6.4$) years. This group had been homeless for an average of 13.6 ($SD = 18.0$) months before entering the study with the longest full-time job lasting an average of 54.2 ($SD = 54.5$) months. Thirty-four percent of the clients were veterans.

Subjects who completed at least one follow-up assessment (131) were compared to those who had no follow-up assessments (45) on demographic and outcome variables at baseline. Subjects with no follow-up revealed significantly fewer positive tests for cocaine at baseline ($p = 0.02$, Chi-Square Test) and reported shorter lifetime marijuana use ($p = 0.03$, Wilcoxon Test) than those who completed at least one follow-up assessment.

Treatment Attendance

Table 1 shows the frequency breakdown of the three attendance groups: Low (less than .5 treatment days per week; $M = .18$; $SD = .015$), Medium (range is .5 to less than 2 treatment days per week; $M = .85$; $SD = .12$), and High (range is 2 to 6.63 treatment days per week; $M = 4.1$; $SD = 1.1$). There were significantly more Usual Care clients in the Low attendance group than Enhanced Care and more Enhanced Care than Usual Care clients in the High attendance group (Chi Square = 41.43, 2 df, $p < 0.0001$). There were no significant differences found between attendance groups on demographic variables, employment history, homelessness, or primary drug of abuse at baseline.

Treatment Attendance and Outcome

Outcome results are presented in four primary areas: days alcohol use in the last 30 days, proportion of positive cocaine urine toxicologies at

TABLE 1. Number and percentages of clients in treatment attendance groups for total sample by intervention group.

Attendance Group	Total (N = 131)	Enhanced Care (n = 69)	Usual Care (n = 62)	p§
Low*	57 (43.5%)	15 (26.3%)	42 (73.7%)	<.001
Medium†	34 (26.0%)	17 (50%)	17 (50%)	
High‡	40 (30.5%)	37 (92.5%)	3 (7.5%)	

*   Low: < .5 contacts per week

†   Medium: .5 to <2 contacts per week

‡   High: 2 to 6.63 contacts per week

§   Chi Square analysis between Enhanced and Usual Care groups versus Treatment Attendance was significant (Chi Square = 41.43, 2 df, $p < .001$).

each assessment point, days homeless in the last 60 days, and days employed in the last 30 days. Figure 1 presents the outcome results in medians (proportions for cocaine toxicologies) as a function of three attendance groups. Wei-Lachin longitudinal analyses[19,20] of treatment outcome as a function of treatment attendance across four time points were conducted and significant differences between attendance groups are presented. For alcohol use, clients in the High attendance group revealed significantly fewer days of alcohol use in the last 30 days than clients in the Low (Wei-Lachin test statistic = 35.0, 4 df, p <0.001) and Medium (Wei-Lachin test statistic = 10.0, 4 df, p = 0.04) attendance groups across time. The High attendance group had significantly fewer positive cocaine toxicologies than both Medium (Wei-Lachin test statistic = 10.4, 4 df, p = 0.03) and Low (Wei-Lachin test statistic = 32.1 , 4 df, p < 0.001) attendance groups across time. High attendance clients revealed fewer days homeless across all time points than the Low (Wei-Lachin test statistic = 17.2, 4 df, p = 0.0002) and Medium (Wei-Lachin test statistic = 9.9, 4 df, p = 0.04) attendance groups. Although the median days employed in the last 30 days appear to be different across the attendance groups, particularly at the 6- and 12-month follow-up points, statistical significance at the .05 level was not reached. There was much variability in this outcome variable with days employed ranging from 0 to 30 days for all attendance groups at all time points. A trend towards statistical significance and certain practical significance is noted.

Table 2 shows significant and non-significant interactions between attendance groups on the outcome variables for each follow-up point. The results show patterns of the effect of attendance on treatment outcome by attendance groups across time. No significant interactions were found between Low versus Medium attendance groups for any of the outcome variables at follow-up, except for alcohol use at the 2-month follow-up point. For Low versus High attendance groups, significant interactions were consistently found for alcohol, cocaine, and homelessness outcome variables at all follow-up points. Significant interactions between Medium versus High groups on the employment variable were found for all follow-up points and at various other time points for the remaining outcome variables.

DISCUSSION

This was a retrospective study of the effect of treatment attendance by clients attending two outpatient substance abuse treatment programs on important treatment outcome variables measured across a one-year period.

FIGURE 1. Longitudinal Analyses of Four Treatment Outcome Variables as a Function of Three Treatment Attendance Groups.

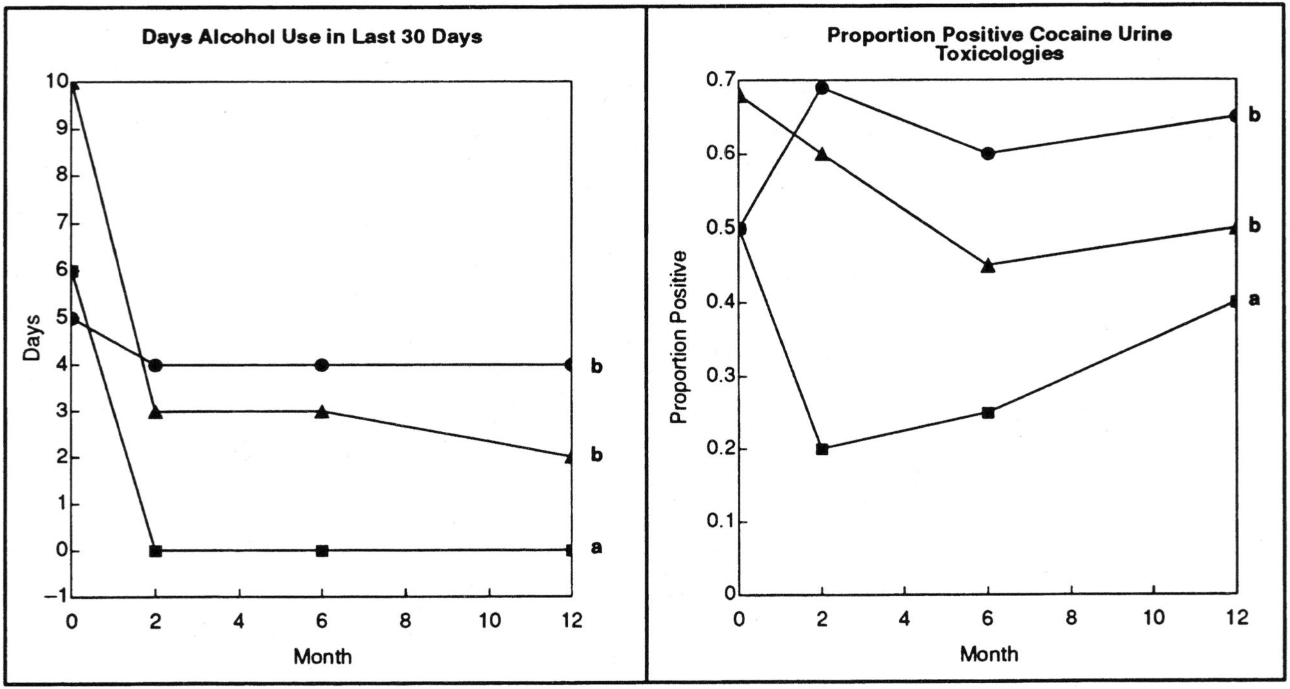

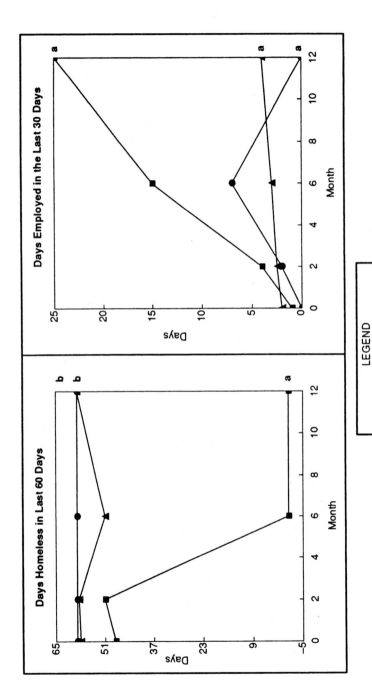

NOTE: Letters (a, b) that differ indicate significantly different medians (proportions for cocaine) between treatment attendance groups across all time points on Wei-Lachin multivariate test ($p < 0.05$).

TABLE 2. Interactions between outcome variables and attendance groups at each follow-up point.

Days Alcohol Use in Last 30 Days

	Attendance Group Comparison		
Time Point	Low vs. Medium	Low vs. High	Medium vs. High
Baseline	NS	NS	NS
2-Month	1.64 p = 0.05	5.16 p < 0.001	2.79 p = 0.003
6-Month	NS	1.64 p = 0.05	NS
12-Month	NS	3.08 p = 0.001	1.88 p = 0.03

Proportion Positive Cocaine Urine Toxicologies

	Attendance Group Comparison		
Time Point	Low vs. Medium	Low vs. High	Medium vs. High
Baseline	NS	NS	NS
2-Month	NS	4.83 p < 0.001	3.18 p = 0.001
6-Month	NS	3.03 p = 0.01	NS
12-Month	NS	1.87 p = 0.031	NS

Days Homeless in Last 60 Days

	Attendance Group Comparison		
Time Point	Low vs. Medium	Low vs. High	Medium vs. High
Baseline	NS	1.80 p = 0.036	NS
2-Month	NS	2.44 p = 0.007	1.87 p = 0.03
6-Month	NS	2.88 p = 0.002	2.40 p = 0.008
12-Month	NS	2.85 p = 0.002	2.24 p = 0.012

Days Employed in the Last 30 Days

	Attendance Group Comparison		
Time Point	Low vs. Medium	Low vs. High	Medium vs. High
Baseline	NS	NS	NS
2-Month	NS	NS	NS
6-Month	NS	NS	− 2.00 p = 0.02
12-Month	NS	− 1.87 p = 0.03	NS

Note: Significant interactions report Wei-Lachin standardized u statistics (1 degree of freedom) and p values. NS = interaction not significant at 0.05 level.

The investigation of the role treatment attendance played on treatment outcome revealed that more attendance during a two-month intensive day treatment program was associated with better long-term outcome. Reductions in alcohol use, cocaine use and homelessness were more likely to occur in clients who received an average of 4.1 days per week (High attendance or Enhanced Care group) than clients who attended less. These results are consistent with the literature suggesting that more intensive treatment during the early phase of treatment results in better treatment outcome with cocaine abusers, but has now been demonstrated with homeless cocaine abusers who have additional problems associated with housing and employment.

These analyses were conducted after analyses comparing two treatment groups: an Enhanced Care day treatment program with Usual Care on the same primary outcome variables presented. The previous comparison of the Enhanced Care with the Usual Care program revealed significant differences favoring day treatment longitudinally over a one-year period for cocaine urine toxicologies, alcohol use, and days homeless.[17] These findings were generally consistent with the findings of the present analyses of outcome as a function of program attendance, in that, the Low attendance group was generally composed of Usual Care clients and the High attendance group consisted mostly of Enhanced Care day treatment clients. This finding suggests that greater attendance and consequently better outcome is more likely to occur in a program that requires more participation than a program that requires less.

Since this was a retrospective study, not a randomized study of treatment attendance, the limitations of this type of investigation should be taken into account. For example, there may be a selection bias operating since subjects were not randomly assigned to treatment attendance groups. Secondly, this was not an a priori hypothesis driven study, thus, exploratory studies of this sort are limited by post hoc hypotheses. Finally, cut off points for the attendance groups were determined arbitrarily according to face valid changes in the distributions and may not be generalizable. The sorting of clients retrospectively into groups based on attendance creates a sample of data that speaks to a possible relationship between client motivation and compliance on subsequent clinical outcome, but is limited in predicting the relationship between planned treatment attendance and subsequent outcome.

The Birmingham Substance Abuse Homeless Project demonstrates the ability of an intensive day treatment program in retaining and successfully treating homeless persons with cocaine abuse.[17] This project was able to retain 74 percent of all homeless clients recruited into the study in some level of treatment and one third of these experienced high levels of treatment attendance or almost daily contact during a two-month outpatient treatment period. While the retention and participation rates fall short of those anticipated in the design, the rates obtained in this study represent successful treatment retention for this population and suggest that intensive day treatment can be successful with homeless persons abusing cocaine if early participation is frequent. It is now important to investigate those characteristics predictive of clients who are more and less likely to stay in treatment and consider ways to improve retention in treatment of homeless persons with substance abuse problems.

REFERENCES

1. Institute of Medicine. Broadening the base of treatment for alcohol problems. Washington, DC: National Academy Press. 1990.

2. Kleinman PH, Woody GE, Todd T, Millman RB, Yang SY, Kemp J, Lippton D. Crack and cocaine abusers in outpatient psychotherapy. NIDA Research Monograph Series. 1990; 104:24-35.

3. Weddington WW, Brown FS, Haeretzen CA, Cone EJ, Dax EM, Herning RI and Michaelson BS. Changes in mood, craving and sleep during short term abstinence reported by male cocaine addicts: A controlled residential study. Archives of General Psychiatry. 1990; 47:861-868.

4. Dole VP, Nyswander ME, Warner A. Successful treatment of 750 criminal addicts. Journal of the American Medical Association.1968; 206:2708-11.

5. Hubbard RL, Marsden ME, Rachal JV, Harwood HS, Cavanaugh ER, Ginzburg HM. Drug abuse treatment: A national study of effectiveness. Chapel Hill: The University of North Carolina Press; 1989.

6. McLellan A, Thomas LL, O'Brien CP, Barr HL, Evans F. Alcohol and drug abuse treatment in three different populations: Is it predictable? American Journal of Drug and Alcohol Abuse. 1986; 12:101-20.

7. Simpson DD. Treatment for drug abuse: Follow-up outcomes and length of time spent. Archives of General Psychiatry. 1981; 38:875-80.

8. Washton AM, Gold MS, Pottash AC. Treatment outcome in cocaine abusers in NIDA Research Monograph 67. Rockville, MD. National Institute on Drug Abuse: 1986.

9. Washton AM, Stone-Washton N. Abstinence and relapse in outpatient cocaine addicts. Journal of Psychoactive Drugs. 1990; 22(2):135-147.

10. Wallace BC. Crack cocaine: A practical treatment approach for the chemically dependent. New York: Brunner/Mazal; 1991.

11. Washton AM. Outpatient treatment techniques. In AM Washton and MS Gold, eds. Cocaine: A Clinicians' handbook. New York: Guilford Press; 1987.

12. Washton AM. Cocaine addiction: Treatment, recovery, and relapse prevention. New York: W.W. Norton; 1989.

13. Washton AM, Stone NS, Hendrickson EC. Cocaine abuse. In DM Donovan and GA Marlatt, eds. Assessment of addictive behaviors. New York: Guilford Press; 1988.

14. O'Brien CP, Alterman A, Walter D, Childress AR, McLellan AT. Evaluation of treatment for cocaine dependence. NIDA Research Monograph 1989; 95: 78-84.

15. Higgins S, Delaney D, Budney A, Bickel WK, Hughes JR, Foerg F, Fenwick KW. A behavioral approach to achieving initial cocaine abstinence. American Journal of Psychiatry. 1991; 148(9):1218-1224.

16. Raczynski JM, Schumacher J, Milby JB, Michael, M, Engle M, Lerner, M and Wooley, T. Comparative substance abuse treatments for the homeless: The Birmingham project. Alcoholism Treatment Quarterly. 1993; 10(3/4):217-233.

17. Milby JB, Schumacher JE, Raczynski JM, Engle M, Caldwell E, Michael M, Carr J. Treatment for homeless cocaine abusers: Retention, process, and outcome. NIDA Research Monograph Series. Problems of Drug Dependence 1994: Proceedings of the 56th Annual Scientific Meeting. The College on Problems of Drug Dependence, Inc. Volume II. 1994:496.

18. American Psychiatric Association. Diagnostic and statistical manual of mental disorders, (third edition revised), Washington, D.C.: American Psychiatric Association; 1987.

19. Wei LJ, and Lachin, JM. Two sample asymptotically distribution-free tests for incomplete multivariate observations. J Am Stat Assn. 1984; 79:6533-661.

20. Wei LJ, and Johnson WE. Combining dependents tests with incomplete repeated measurements. Biometrika. 1985; 72:359-364.

21. Davis CS. Semi-parametric and non-parametric methods for the analysis of repeated measurements with applications to clinical trials. Statistics in Medicine. 1991; 10:1959-1980.

Effective Services
for Homeless Substance Abusers

G. Nicholas Braucht, PhD
Charles S. Reichardt, PhD
Lisa J. Geissler, PhD
Carol A. Bormann, PhD
Carol F. Kwiatkowski, PhD
Michael W. Kirby, Jr., PhD

SUMMARY. A heterogeneous and representative sample of 323 homeless individuals in the metropolitan-Denver area with alcohol or other substance abuse problems received a comprehensive array of substance-abuse treatment services. Following treatment, these individuals showed dramatic improvement on average in their (a) levels of alcohol and drug use, (b) housing status, (c) physical and mental health, (d) employment, and (e) quality of life. Those who received more service improved more than those who received less service. These improvements are attributable, at least partly, to the treatment rather than to alternative hypotheses such as spontaneous remission.

G. Nicholas Braucht, Charles S. Reichardt, Lisa J. Geissler, Carol A. Bormann, and Carol F. Kwiatkowski are affiliated with the Department of Psychology, University of Denver.

Michael W. Kirby, Jr., is affiliated with the Arapahoe House.

Address correspondence to either G. Nicholas Braucht or Charles S. Reichardt, Department of Psychology, University of Denver, Denver, CO 80208.

We would like to thank the editors for their helpful comments.

Preparation of this manuscript was supported, in part, by Grant U01-AA08778 from the National Institute on Alcohol Abuse and Alcoholism.

[Haworth co-indexing entry note]: "Effective Services for Homeless Substance Abusers." Braucht, Nicholas G., et al. Co-published simultaneously in the *Journal of Addictive Diseases* (The Haworth Medical Press, an imprint of The Haworth Press, Inc.) Vol. 14, No. 4, 1995, pp. 87-109; and: *The Effectiveness of Social Interventions for Homeless Substance Abusers* (ed: Gerald J. Stahler) The Haworth Medical Press, an imprint of The Haworth Press, Inc., 1995, pp. 87-109. Single or multiple copies of this article are available from The Haworth Document Delivery Service [1-800-342-9678; 9:00 a.m. - 5:00 p.m. (EST)].

However, the rate of improvement generally slowed during the six-month follow-up period.

A random half of the clients received intensive case management in addition to the other services. Case management marginally increased clients' contacts with addictions counselors, but had little effect on the level of other services received or on the tailoring of services to client needs. As a result, case management also had little, if any, effect on outcomes. *[Article copies available from The Haworth Document Delivery Service: 1-800-342-9678.]*

INTRODUCTION

During the past decade, research on homeless individuals in this country has shown that contemporary homelessness is substantially associated with alcohol and other drug problems[1-4] and that homeless persons with substance abuse problems are at elevated risk for multiple additional problems, including psychiatric disorders, physical health problems, and employment problems.[5-9] Not only do contemporary homeless substance abusers appear to be a quite heterogeneous group with multiple interrelated problems and a wide spectrum of service needs, but they also appear to face a welter of potential barriers to service delivery and access.[10] In addition, it is difficult for any one service system to address the variety of problems, needs, and barriers to access posed by contemporary homeless substance abusers.

To address the multifaceted problems presented by homeless substance abusers, a service delivery strategy based upon a dyadic case management model was developed and implemented at Arapahoe House, which is the largest not-for-profit substance abuse treatment center in Colorado and the largest contractor to the Alcohol and Drug Abuse Division of the Colorado Department of Health. Separate from the case management model that was developed specifically for the present research project, Arapahoe House also has long offered a comprehensive array of substance abuse treatment and rehabilitation services, including detoxification, residential and outpatient services, substance abuse counseling, literacy and vocational assessment, and job training and placement.

The particular model of case management that was implemented at Arapahoe House for the present project is described in detail elsewhere.[11] In brief, the case management model was one in which case managers worked in pairs (dyads) with a caseload averaging 15 clients per dyad (and never exceeding 17 clients per dyad) and with a consequent high intensity of client contact *in situ*, rather than in a centralized office location. The dyadic structure was adopted to enhance the continuity of service delivery (even in the face of case manager turnover, illness, and vacations), and to ensure that each case manager had a partner who could both provide support and bring complementary perspectives, experience, and skills to the task of managing the delivery of services to each client. This dyadic and intensive case management model was explicitly designed to identify the individual service needs of each client, to match these needs with the most appropriate agency or service regardless of location, and to provide continuity of case manager contact and service delivery over a period of time. Building upon the general tradition of social case work, this dyadic case management model emphasized the importance of proactive outreach, client identification and assessment, development of an individually-tailored and comprehensive service plan for each client, establishment of linkages between service systems and clients such that services were matched to client needs, continuity of service utilization monitoring, and assertive advocacy with community agencies on behalf of clients.[12-19]

Over the course of the study that is reported herein, 323 homeless individuals with alcohol or other substance abuse problems were admitted to Arapahoe House and assessed both before and after treatment on a range of measures including (a) levels of alcohol and other drug use, (b) residential stability, (c) physical health, (d) mental health, (e) employment, and (f) quality of life. All 323 clients had access to the full range of traditional services offered by Arapahoe House. In addition, a random half of the clients received intensive case management. The purpose of the research project was to assess the effectiveness of both Arapahoe House services in general and intensive case management in particular. The results of each of these two assessments are presented separately below. We first discuss the delivery and effectiveness of Arapahoe House services in general, and then the delivery and effectiveness of intensive case management.

STUDY PARTICIPANTS

The 323 participants in the study were drawn from the population of substance abusers who were referred to Arapahoe House for treatment between April 1, 1991 and June 6, 1992. Referral sources included local drop-in centers, homeless shelters, other community sites, public and private agencies, and self-referrals. To be eligible for the study, clients had to meet the following criteria: (1) have no medical or psychiatric problems that would preclude receiving services from Arapahoe House; (2) show evidence of a substance abuse problem; (3) be homeless; (4) be 18 years old or older; (5) be likely to remain in the metro area for the duration of the study; (6) be willing to participate in the study; and (7) be willing to participate in residential treatment through Arapahoe House.

Because of extensive outreach efforts, the pool of potential study participants who were screened for eligibility was believed to consist of virtually the entire population of homeless substance abusers in the Denver metropolitan area who were willing to receive services for substance abuse and homelessness. Of the 1,425 individuals in this population, 668 met the eligibility criteria and 323 were admitted to the study. The selection of the 323 clients from the eligible pool of 668 was based solely on whether there was room for the client in the study at the time the client was referred for treatment.

Background characteristics of the sample of 323 clients in the study, as assessed at baseline, are presented in Table 1. A client with a composite of the most typical characteristics would be a 35-year-old, caucasian male who has been previously married, has children, has been homeless for 3 years, has graduated from high school, has a profession, skill or trade, and has a substance abuse problem with alcohol. However, there was substantial heterogeneity in the sample of clients. For example, 15% of the sample were women, 29% were African-Americans, 10% were Hispanic, 38% had drug problems either in addition to or in place of alcohol problems, and 20% had a lifetime Axis I psychiatric diagnosis. As Table 4 reveals, 74% of the study clients reported alcohol as their primary substance of abuse. Another 24% reported that cocaine or crack was their primary substance of abuse. Only 2% (7 out of 323 clients) reported some other drug (besides alcohol or cocaine/crack) as their primary substance of abuse.

PROCEDURES

Study clients were assessed at three points in time. Upon referral to Arapahoe House, study clients were placed in a transitional residence for 3 to 5 days, during which time they received detoxification services as needed. The first (or baseline) assessment occurred during the stay in the transitional residence. Following their stay in the transitional residence, clients were enrolled in either residential or outpatient treatment at Arapahoe House for four months. The second (or Time 2) assessment took place at the time of discharge from Arapahoe House, which was at the end of the four-month treatment period. The third (or Time 3) assessment took place six months after discharge (i.e., ten months after the baseline assessment).

A range of outcome measures was collected at each of the three assessment points. The present report focuses on 17 outcome measures, which span 10 different substantive domains. These 17 outcome measures were selected because they were the most central measures within each of the 10 substantive domains. Table 2 presents the mean and standard deviation at baseline for each of the 17 outcome measures. Those measures for which desired change is in the positive direction are bold-faced. This convention is also used in the tables that follow.

In 7 of the 10 substantive domains, we have chosen a pair of outcome measures for presentation in the present report. The correlation at baseline between these pairs of outcome measures within each of the substantive domains are reported in the right-hand column of Table 2. Except for the correlation between the two measures of social relations, these correlations are all quite high in absolute value, and suggest that the measures have reasonable reliability. In contrast, the correlations of the outcome measures across the 10 substantive domains at baseline are relatively low. Except for the correlation between "General Satisfaction with Life" and "Satisfaction with Family Situation" which was .43 ($p < .01$), none of the correlations was greater than 0.4 in absolute value, and the majority were less than 0.2. These relatively low correlations reflect substantial discriminant validity among the 10 substantive domains.

SERVICES RECEIVED

Once admitted to Arapahoe House, the 323 study clients had access to the complete array of treatment and rehabilitation services offered by Arapahoe House. On average, the 323 study clients spent 8 days (with a standard deviation, SD, of 4 days) in the Arapahoe House detoxification facility during the four-month treatment period and 2 days (SD = 3) in the detoxification facility during the six-month follow-up period. In addition, the 323 study participants spent an average of 26 days (SD = 24) in residence in Arapahoe House facilities (excluding the detoxification facility) during the four-month treatment period and 3 days (SD = 13) in residence during the six-month follow-up period. On average, the 323 study participants also had 105 contacts (SD = 62) with an addictions counselor during the four-month treatment period and 3 contacts (SD = 16) during the six-month follow-up period. During the four-month treatment period, study clients reported receiving on average an additional 41 hours (SD = 72) of substance-abuse treatment and 64 days (SD = 32) of housing from agencies other than Arapahoe House. The preceding results on services received from Arapahoe House are based on internal records from Arapahoe House and are calculated across the entire sample of 323 clients because data were available for the entire sample. The preceding results on services received from agencies other than Arapahoe House are based on self-report inter-

TABLE 1. Backgroud Characteristics of the 323 Study Clients.

The Results Presented are either Percentages or Means
(with Standard Deviations in Parantheses)

Gender:
   Males   85%
   Females   15%

Age in Years: 35.4   (8.3)

Ethnicity:
   Caucasian   56%
   African-American   29%
   Hispanic   10%
   Native American   4%
   Other/Missing   1%

Alcohol Abuse:
   Alchohol is Primary Substance of Abuse   74%
   Have Alcohol Problems   82%
   Number of Years of Alcohol Use   14.4   (9.4)
   Number of Times in Alcohol Abuse Treatment   15.2   (26.8)

Drug Abuse:
   Have Drug Problems   38%
   Number of Years of Drug Use   7.5   (7.4)
   Number of Times in Drug Abuse Treatment   1.1   (3.0)

Homelessness:
   Years Homeless   3.3   (4.6)
   Number of Times Homeless   9.7   (22.8)
   Years Living in Metro Area   13.2   (12.8)
   Age First Became Homeless   28.3   (9.6)

   Days in the Last 60 Spent in:
      Someone Else's Apartment/House   11.9   (17.2)
      On Street or Other Outdoor Place   11.0   (16.4)
      Emergency Shelter   9.0   (15.6)

Education and Employment:
   Years of Education   12.1   (2.1)
   Years at Longest Full Time Job   3.9   (4.2)
   Usually Employed Full Time in Past Year   31%
   Have a Profession, Trade or Skill   77%

   Profession, Trade, or Skill:
     1. Higher Executives & Major Professionals   1%
     2. Business Managers & Lesser Professionals   5%
     3. Admin. Personnel & Minor Professionals   11%
     4. Clerical/Sales Personnel & Technicians   9%
     5. Skilled Manual Laborers   27%
     6. Semi-Skilled and Machine Operators   19%
     7. Unskilled Personnel   6%
     8. No Profession, Trade, or Skill   23%

Medical and Mental Health:
Have Chronic Medical Problems	19%	
Lifetime Number of Overnight Hospital Stays	3.4	(5.0)
Ever Had Lifetime Axis I Diagnosis	20%	
Ever Had Lifetime Axis II Diagnosis	24%	
Ever Had Psychiatric Hospitalization	19%	
Ever Had Psychiatric Outpatient Treatment	20%	
Ever Been Prescribed Psychiatric Medications	20%	
Ever Attempted Suicide	26%	

Legal History:
Lifetime Number of Arrests	5.3	(9.4)
Lifetime Number of Months in Jail	18.0	(34.5)

Social and Family Relationships:
Marital Status:
Married/Remarried	3%	
Widowed/Divorced/Separated	54%	
Never Married	44%	
Have Any Children	57%	
Number of Close Relationships	4.3	(2.0)
Number of Problematic Relationships	2.5	(2.3)

Satisfied with Marital Status:
Yes	47%
Indifferent	16%
No	37%

Usual Living Arrangement in Last Year:
With Others	35%
Alone	33%
No Stable Arrange or Controlled Environment	32%

Victimization:
Physical Abuse by Someone Known	38%
Sexual Abuse by Someone Known	13%
Ever Assaulted	61%
Ever Robbed	63%

views conducted at the Time 2 (i.e., the four-month) assessment and are calculated across the 301 (out of the 323) clients for whom these specific self-report data were available.

CHANGES OVER TIME

Table 3 reports the means and mean percentage changes on the 17 outcome measures at baseline, Time 2 and Time 3. Of the 323 clients who were admitted to the study, 6% could not be found for the Time 2 assessment, and 12% could not be found for the Time 3 assessment. If data on a variable were not available for an individual at one or more of the three

TABLE 2. Means, Standard Deviations, and Correlations of 17 Outcome Measures at Baseline.

	Direction of Desired Change	Mean	Standard Deviation	Correlation between Variable Pairs
Alcohol Use				
Number of Days in Last 30 that Used Alcohol	–	18.85	10.46	
Alcohol Use Problems Composite	–	0.59	0.28	.82[†]
(0 = no problems, 1 = most problems)				
Drug Use				
Number of Days in Last 30 that Used Drugs	–	7.83	10.75	
Drug Use Problems Composite	–	0.11	0.14	.90[†]
(0 = no problems, 1 = most problems)				
Employment				
Number of Days in Last 30 that Paid for Working	+	4.72	6.40	
Employment Problems Composite	–	0.83	0.18	–.51[†]
(0 = no problems, 1 = most problems)				
Housing Status				
Number of Days in Last 60 Not Literally Homeless	+	32.48	21.54	
Quality of Housing During the Last 60 Days	+	7.07	2.45	.79[†]
(1 = low quality, 14 = high quality)				

Illegal Activities				
Seriousness of Present Legal Problems (0 = not at all, 4 = extremely)	−	0.63	1.20	
Legal Problems Composite (0 = no problems, 1 = most problems)	−	0.13	0.19	.83†
Life Satisfaction				
General Satisfaction with Life (1 = terrible, 7 = delighted)	+	2.70	1.48	
Living Skills				
Problems with Living Skills (0 = no problem, 48 = serious problem)	−	21.99	6.33	
Mental Health				
Psychological Problems Composite (0 = good, 1 = poor)	−	0.28	0.23	
Physical Health				
Number of Days in Last 30 with Medical Problems	−	5.59	9.94	
Medical Problems Composite (0 = no problems, 1 = most problems)	−	0.22	0.30	.85†
Social Relations				
Satisfaction with Family Situation (1 = terrible, 7 = delighted)	+	3.39	1.74	
Personal Conflicts Composite	−	0.25	0.21	−.17†

† $p < .01$

TABLE 3. Percentage Change in the 17 Outcome Measures.

	N†	Time1 Mean	Time2 Mean	Time3 Mean	Percent Mean Change from Time1 to Time2	p‡	Percent Mean Change from Time1 to Time3	p‡	Percent Mean Change from Time2 to Time3	p‡
Alcohol Use										
Alcohol Use	282	18.95	7.87	7.53	−58.5	<.001	−60.3	<.001	−4.3	.586
Alcohol Composite	282	0.59	0.28	0.23	−53.7	<.001	−61.6	<.001	−17.1	.006
Drug Use										
Drug Use	282	7.76	2.34	3.04	−69.8	<.001	−60.8	<.001	29.9	.182
Drug Composite	282	0.11	0.05	0.04	−58.4	<.001	−65.5	<.001	−17.0	.198
Employment										
Employment Paid	278	4.76	11.75	10.66	146.8	<.001	124.0	<.001	−9.3	.104
Employ. Composite	282	0.83	0.73	0.72	−12.2	<.001	−13.8	<.001	−1.8	.251
Housing Status										
Housing Days	274	33.49	49.91	52.80	49.0	<.001	57.7	<.001	5.8	.006
Housing Quality	274	7.14	8.86	9.53	24.1	<.001	33.5	<.001	7.6	<.001
Illegal Activities										
Legal Problems	271	0.68	0.56	0.53	−18.4	.139	−22.3	.099	−4.7	.770
Legal Composite	282	0.13	0.10	0.08	−22.4	.020	−37.3	<.001	−19.2	.110

	N				%	p	%	p	%	p
Life Satisfaction										
Life Satisfaction	201	2.76	4.09	4.26	48.2	<.001	54.3	<.001	4.2	.197
Living Skills										
Living Skills	200	21.84	17.90	16.81	−18.0	<.001	−23.0	<.001	−6.1	.011
Mental Health										
Psych. Composite	279	0.28	0.18	0.11	−35.9	<.001	−60.1	<.001	−37.8	<.001
Physical Health										
Medical Problems	279	5.76	5.26	4.25	−8.7	.491	−26.2	.044	−19.2	.181
Medical Composite	279	0.23	0.21	0.16	−6.2	.542	−30.5	.003	−25.9	.023
Social Relations										
Family Satisfaction	199	3.35	3.96	4.13	18.2	<.001	23.3	<.001	4.3	.157
Social Composite	281	0.25	0.16	0.14	−34.1	<.001	−44.6	<.001	−15.9	.071

† N is the number of clients on which the statistics in each row are based. If data were not available for an individual at one or more of the three assessments in a given row, data from that individual were not included for the calculations in that row.

‡ p is the obtained-p value for a two-tailed, matched-pairs t test of the mean changes over time.

Change in an undesirable direction is underlined.

TABLE 4. Comparisons of High- and Low-Service Groups.

	Baseline		Time 2		Baseline by Time 2 Interaction p¶	Time 3		Baseline by Time 3 Interaction p¶
	Desired Direction†	p§	Desired Direction‡	p§		Desired Direction‡	p§	
Alcohol Use								
Alcohol Use	YES	.007	YES	.036	.000	YES	.344	.004
Alcohol Composite	YES	.001	YES	.085	.000	YES	.611	.002
Drug Use								
Drug Use	NO	.083	YES	.001	.743	YES	.132	.733
Drug Composite	NO	.167	YES	.001	.366	YES	.581	.394
Employment								
Employment Paid	NO	.355	YES	.000	.000	YES	.012	.044
Employ. Composite	NO	.011	YES	.000	.047	YES	.008	.215
Housing Status								
Housing Days	NO	.628	YES	.006	.092	YES	.585	.955
Housing Quality	NO	.421	YES	.056	.380	YES	.162	.459
Illegal Activities								
Legal Problems	YES	.776	YES	.498	.422	YES	.252	.133
Legal Composite	YES	.526	YES	.084	.043	YES	.227	.087

Measure	Baseline†	p§	Time 2‡	p§	p¶	Time 3‡	p§	p¶
Life Satisfaction								
Life Satisfaction	YES	.147	YES	.006	.001	YES	.671	.075
Living Skills								
Living Skills	YES	.035	YES	.263	.007	NO	.075	.573
Mental Health								
Psych. Composite	NO	.744	YES	.025	.131	YES	.509	.740
Physical Health								
Medical Problems	YES	.528	NO	.458	.955	YES	.641	.301
Medical Composite	NO	.353	YES	.718	.646	YES	.533	.898
Social Relations								
Family Satisfaction	YES	.708	YES	.529	.802	YES	.899	.941
Social Composite	NO	.304	YES	.121	.726	NO	.940	.455

† At baseline, the "desired direction" arises when the mean level of problems is higher, or the mean level of functioning is lower, for the low-service group than for the high-service group. In other words, it is desirable if those who need more services get more services.

‡ At Time 2 and Time 3, the "desired direction" arises when the high-service group had a lower mean level of problems or a higher mean level of functioning than the low-service group. In other words, it is desirable if those who received more services had fewer problems after treatment than those who received fewer services.

§ p is the obtained-p level for an independent-groups t test of the mean differences between the high-service and low-service groups.

¶ p is the obtained-p level for a test of the interaction between the group (high-service and low-service) and the time of measurement (baseline and Time 2 or Time 3) in a repeated-measures analysis of variance.

assessments, data from that individual were not included in the results for that variable for any of the three time points in Table 3. The column labeled "N" in Table 3 reports the number of clients on which the statistics in each row are based and the columns labeled "p" in Table 3 report the obtained-p values for matched-paired t tests of the mean changes over time.

For 14 of the 17 outcome measures, the mean change from baseline to Time 2 was statistically significant. In addition, the direction of the mean change from baseline to Time 2 was in the desired direction on all 17 outcome measures, which means that study clients were better functioning or had fewer problems at Time 2 than at baseline on all 17 measures. The percentage mean changes ranged in size from 6% to 146%, and mean changes on 9 of the 17 measures were larger than 30%.

The mean changes from baseline to Time 3 were in the desired direction for all 17 outcome measures and were statistically significant on 16 of the 17 measures. Twelve out of the 17 measures showed percentage mean changes of 30% or more. In addition, fifteen of the 17 mean changes from Time 2 to Time 3 were in the desired direction. The percentage mean changes on the two variables ("Drug Use" and "Employment Paid") that were in the undesired directions are underlined in Table 3. However, on only 6 of the 17 measures were the mean changes from Time 2 to Time 3 statistically significant at the .05 level, though these 6 were all in the desired direction. Only 1 out of 17 percentage mean changes from Time 2 to Time 3 was greater than 30%.

In summary, very substantial improvement occurred on most outcome measures from baseline to Time 2. For the most part, improvement continued from Time 2 to Time 3, though the change was less than from baseline to Time 2. This pattern of change is compatible with the pattern of services received from Arapahoe House over the ten-month period of the study. That is, study clients received substantial amounts of services during the four-month treatment period from baseline to Time 2 but many fewer services during the six-month follow-up period from Time 2 to Time 3.

However, the pattern of change in Table 3 is also compatible with regression toward the mean or spontaneous remission. That is, clients might have been at a low ebb in their functioning when they entered the study and would have regressed back to a higher level of functioning even without receiving treatment. To distinguish between these two potential explanations (i.e., a treatment effect versus regression to the mean), we divided the study clients as equally as possible into two groups based on the number of days in residence at Arapahoe House. This produced a high-service group ($N = 190$) that averaged 38 days in residence and 145 contacts with addictions counselors and a low-service group ($N = 133$) that averaged only 9 days in residence and only 50 contacts with addictions counselors.

The first column of results in Table 4 reveals whether the mean difference between the high-service and low-service groups was in the "desired direction" at baseline on each of the 17 outcome measures. At baseline, being in the "desired direction" means that those who needed more services received more services (i.e., the mean level of problems at baseline was higher, or the mean level of functioning at baseline was lower, for the high-service group than for the low-service group). In other words, it would have been desirable for more services to go to those in greater need. The first column reveals that this desired pattern occurred on only 8 of the 17 outcome measures. The next column in Table 4 reports the obtained-p level for an independent-groups *t* test of the mean difference between the high-service and low-service groups at baseline for each variable.

The next two columns in Table 4 give similar results for Time 2, though the definition of the "desired direction" changes. At Time 2, being in the "desired direction" means that those who received a greater number of services had a lower mean level of problems or a higher mean level of functioning at Time 2 than those who received fewer services. In other words, it would be desirable for those who received a greater number of services to have had fewer problems after treatment than those who received fewer services. This was the case for all but one of the 17 outcome measures. This is consistent with the hypothesis that the treatment is effective. The obtained-p level for an independent-groups *t* test of the mean difference between the high-service and low-service groups at Time 2 is also given for each variable in Table 4. In addition, the column in Table 4 labeled "Baseline by Time 2 Interaction" gives the obtained-p level for a test of the interaction between the group (high-service and low-service) and the time of measurement (baseline and Time 2) in a repeated-measures analysis of variance.

The last three columns of results in Table 4 (just to the right of the double vertical lines) are parallel to the columns of results described in the preceding paragraph; the only difference is that Time 2 has been replaced by Time 3. In other words, one of these columns reports whether the mean difference between the high-service and low-service groups was in the desired direction at Time 3 and one of the columns reports the obtained-p level for an independent-groups *t* test of this mean difference. As at Time 2, a mean difference at Time 3 is in the desired direction if the high-service group had a higher mean level of functioning (or a lower mean level of problems) than the low-service group. Again, this is called the desired direction because it is consistent with the treatment being effective. The mean difference is in the desired direction at Time 3 for all but 2 of the 17 outcome measures. The last column in Table 4 gives the obtained-p level for a test of the interaction between group (high-service and low-service) and the time of measurement (baseline and Time 3) in a repeated-measures analysis of variance.

Overall, the results in Table 4 strongly suggest that the mean change on many of the 17 outcome measures was due at least partly to the services received and not just to regression toward the mean. For example, the first row of Table 4 reveals that there was a crossover interaction between the high-service and low-service groups and time of measurement from baseline to Time 2 on the outcome measure of alcohol use during the last 30 days (i.e., "Alcohol Use"). A picture of this interaction is presented in Figure 1 and shows that the high-service group averaged more days of alcohol use than the low-service group at baseline, but fewer days of alcohol use than the low-service group at Time 2. (This means that the differences were in the desired direction at both baseline and Time 2.) The results in Table 4 show that this crossover interaction is statistically significant (and that the mean differences between the high-service and low-service groups was statistically significant both at baseline and at Time 2). This pattern of results cannot be explained as a consequence of regression toward the mean. Regression toward the mean can account for both groups getting better over time, but can't account for the high-service group starting out worse and ending up better than the low-service group. The most plausible explanation for this cross-over pattern of results is that the greater amount of services received by the high-service group caused a greater reduction in alcohol use than the lesser amount of services received by the low-service group. Note that the crossover interaction from baseline to Time 3 is also statistically significant for alcohol use.

As can be seen in Table 4, the "Alcohol Composite," "Legal Composite," "Life Satisfaction," and "Living Skills" outcome measures also exhibit statistically significant, crossover interactions between the high-service and low-service groups and the time of measurement from baseline to Time 2. In addition, for each of these measures, the high-service group exhibited lower functioning than the low-service group at baseline, but higher functioning than the low-service group at Time 2. Again, none of these interactions can be explained by regression toward the mean. They are all more plausibly explained as effects of the services the clients received. In addition, the crossover interaction from baseline to Time 3 is statistically significant for the "Alcohol Composite" measure.

In addition, both the "Employment Composite" and the outcome measure of the number of days paid for working in the last 30 ("Employment

FIGURE 1. Number of Days in Last 30 that Used Alcohol (Alcohol Use)

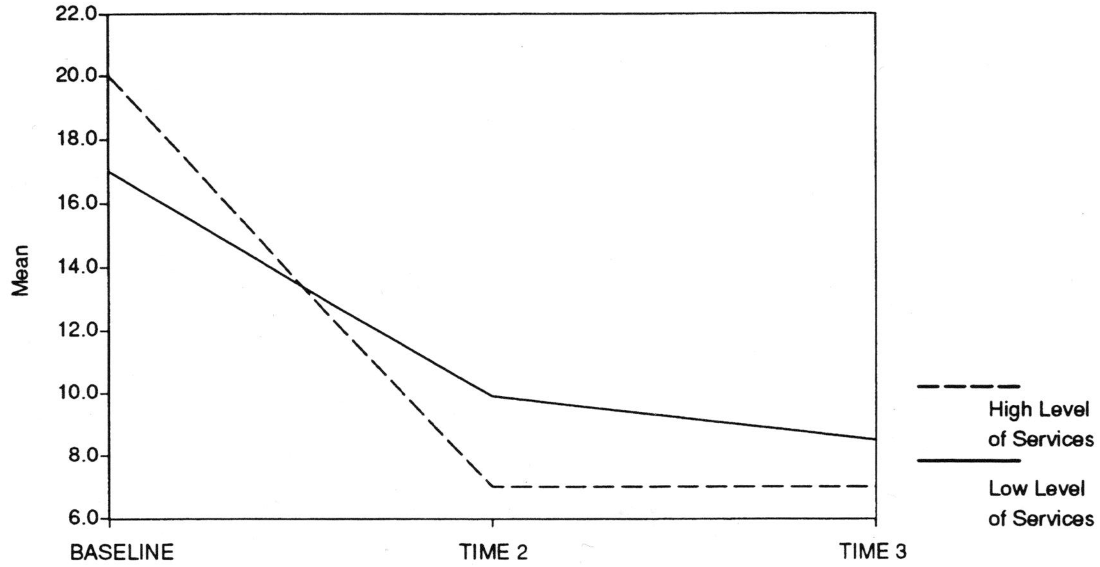

Paid") have statistically significant interactions between group (high-service and low-service) and time of measurement from baseline to Time 2 (and one interaction is significant at Time 3 as well). Though these interactions are not crossover interactions, the data patterns are more plausibly explained as treatment effects than as regression toward the mean. This is because regression toward the mean would predict that the more deviant group at the start would change the most over time. Yet for these two outcome measures, the high-service group is less deviant than the low-service group at baseline but nonetheless changes the most. In addition, using an alternative grouping for the high- and low-services categorization (i.e., grouping on the basis of the number of addictions counselor contacts rather than on the number of days in residence), a statistically significant crossover interaction was obtained for the "Employment Paid" outcome measure ($p < .001$).

Neither of the two outcome measures of drug use produced statistically significant interactions using the high-service and low-service grouping reported in Table 4 (i.e., based on the number of days in residence), but the alternative grouping of the high-service and low-service groups (based on the number of addictions counselor contacts) did produce statistically significant interactions for both of these outcome measures. The same was almost true for the outcome measure of the number of non-homeless days in the last 60 ("Housing Days"); the alternative grouping produced an interaction that just barely missed statistical significance ($p = .052$).

INTENSIVE CASE MANAGEMENT

The 323 study clients were randomly assigned either to a control group ($N = 160$) or an experimental group ($N = 163$). Both of these groups of clients had access to the full array of services offered by Arapahoe House. However, the clients in the experimental group also received intensive case management (ICM) during their four-month treatment periods, while the clients in the control condition did not receive case management.

The Case-Management Model. As noted above, a dyadic and intensive case management model was implemented at Arapahoe House and was designed to ensure that the types and amounts of services needed by each individual client were obtained in a timely and continuous fashion. Case managers were specifically trained to broker the delivery of services within Arapahoe House and to link clients to services from agencies outside of Arapahoe House. Because all the clients in the study were enrolled in treatment at Arapahoe House, the case managers were not trained to act as a client's primary counselor. Nonetheless, case managers were encouraged to provide one-on-one services such as crisis intervention and transportation, as needed. In these ways, case managers both assisted clients directly and brokered the delivery of services by others. Each client in the experimental (ICM) condition received intensive case management services during the four-month treatment period or until the client was discharged from Arapahoe House.

Initial Equivalence and Attrition. Random assignment procedures are often corrupted in practice. The random assignment of clients to the experimental (ICM) and control groups in the present study was implemented with a computer program specifically designed to protect the integrity of the assignment process.[20] Using this computerized procedure, we found no signs of corruption, and the differences between the groups at baseline strongly suggest that the groups were randomly equivalent (i.e., statistically significant mean differences between the ICM and control groups at the .05 level arose on only 7 [3%] out of the 213 quantitative baseline measures).

We also found no evidence that differential attrition introduced meaningful nonequivalence between the groups. We were unable to track 10% and 13% of the control group at Times 2 and 3, respectively, and 4% and 12% of the experimental (ICM) group at these time points. These differences in attrition between the two groups were not statistically significant ($\chi^2[1] = 1.02$ and 0.16, p = .31 and .69, for Times 2 and 3, respectively). In addition, the above described pattern of small and overwhelmingly nonsignificant mean differences between the ICM and control groups on the baseline measures was substantively the same whether we examined the data on all 323 study clients or only on those we were able to track.

Services Received. On average, the experimental (ICM) group clients had 38 service contacts with a case manager during the four-month treatment period and 5 contacts with a case manager during the six-month follow-up period (though there was supposed to be zero contacts during the latter period). The control group clients had no contacts with a case manager during either of these periods.

It was expected that the case managers would substantially increase the amount of services that the clients in the ICM group received from both Arapahoe House and other agencies. This was not the case. For example, the ICM group had, on average, only 12 (about 10%) more contacts with addictions counselors from Arapahoe House than did the control group during the four-month treatment period and less than one additional contact on average during the six-month follow-up period (neither of these differences was statistically significant, $t(298) = 1.62$, $p = .106$ and $t(281) = .29$, $p = .772$, respectively). In addition, the ICM and control groups spent virtually the same average number of days in residence at Arapahoe House (both in detoxification and in other residential facilities). Nor were there any substantively or statistically significant differences between the ICM and control groups in the mean number of self-reported services received or days spent in residence at agencies other than Arapahoe House.

It was also expected that case management would improve the fit between the clients' needs and the services they received. That is, it was expected that services would be better tailored to individual client needs because of ICM. However, the data provided only marginal support for this hypothesis. In particular, the data suggested that case managers may have altered the distribution of days in residence, as compared to the control condition, on the basis of family situation and medical problems so that those clients who were worse off at baseline spent more days in residence and those who were better off at baseline spent fewer days in residence. But these were not dramatic effects, and they were not statistically significant for other types of services or for other baseline measures of need. In addition, within the ICM group, the number of contacts that clients had with case managers was not strongly correlated with the number of other services received either from Arapahoe House or other agencies. For example, the number of contacts that clients had with case managers during the four-month treatment period was correlated .19 ($p < .05$) with the number of contacts the clients had with addictions counselors at Arapahoe House during the four-month treatment period, and .10 ($p > .05$) with the number of days in residence at Arapahoe House during the four-month treatment period.

Effects of ICM on the Outcome Measures. Given that case management appeared to have little effect on the delivery of services to clients (as described immediately above), it is not surprising that ICM appeared to have little effect on outcomes. For example, at Time 2, the mean difference between the ICM and control groups was statistically significant on only 2 out of the 17 outcome measures. The mean difference on one measure (drug use during the last 30 days) favored the ICM group (by 1.5 days), but the difference on the other outcome measure (general life satisfaction) favored the control group. In addition, the majority of the (nonsignificant) mean differences on the other 15 outcome measures favored the control group. No mean difference between the two treatment groups was statistically significant at Time 3. These results were not meaningfully altered with the use of more powerful statistical techniques such as analysis of covariance or multivariate analysis of variance.

DISCUSSION

On average, the 323 study clients received substantial amounts of services from Arapahoe House and other agencies, including residential treatment and addictions counseling. On average, study clients also exhibited dramatic and statistically significant improvements over time in all 10 outcome domains. On most measures, the improvements were larger from baseline to Time 2 than from Time 2 to Time 3. This corresponded to the delivery of services, which was substantially greater from baseline to Time 2 than from Time 2 to Time 3.

In addition, on most outcomes, individuals who received more service improved more than individuals who received less service. These patterns of differential improvement cannot be explained by regression toward the mean or spontaneous remission, but are plausibly attributed to the effects of the services received. In particular, the results support the conclusion that improvements in alcohol use, drug use, employment status, housing status, legal issues, living skills, and life satisfaction were due at least in part to the effects of the services that were delivered by Arapahoe House. Nonetheless, it is important to recognize that these effects were greatest at the end of the four-month treatment period (during which time substantial amounts of services were received) and tended to be smaller six months later (during which time relatively few services were received). This pattern is consistent with the view that the problems faced by homeless substance abusers are chronic in nature and that, while they can be alleviated by treatment, the greatest improvements will be obtained only if treatment continues.

As expected, study clients in the experimental (ICM) condition had a substantial number of contacts with case managers on average, while clients in the control condition had no contact with case managers. However, case management only slightly increased the number of contacts that clients had with addictions counselors. And case management did not appear to substantially influence the amounts of other services received nor the tailoring of services to client needs. As a result, case management had little, if any, demonstrable effect on the outcome measures.

An adequate test of the effectiveness of case management requires both a full and robust supply of services that can be accessed by clients and their case managers, and an implementation of case management that is full and robust. Both of these criteria were met in the present study. The array of services that was available to study clients was extensive and was extensively utilized by the study clients. Case management was also implemented vigorously and comprehensively. In addition, the study clients were a representative and heterogeneous sample of homeless individuals with alcohol or other substance abuse problems. The study clients exhibited substantial and chronic psychological and physical needs that well justified their receiving intensive services from Arapahoe House and other agencies. As a result, we believe the present study was a fair test of the effectiveness of case management as implemented over a four-month period of time (though one might argue that an adequate test of case management would require a longer treatment period than four months).

However, as in all studies, the results of the present project are constrained by the context. Having a full array of services available to study clients might be a double-edged sword for case management. On the one hand, case managers by themselves can have little effect if adequate services for treating clients are not available. But at the same time, case managers can perhaps have little effect in an environment where services are plentiful and easily accessed by clients without much assistance. The latter type of environment was present at Arapahoe House. Even without case management, clients in the control condition received very substantial amounts of services. Perhaps case management would be shown to be more effective in a context, unlike Arapahoe House, where services are available but not easily accessible without a case manager's assistance.

REFERENCES

1. Fischer PJ, Breakey WR. Homelessness and mental health: An overview. Int J of Mental Health. 1986; 14:6-41.

2. Fischer PJ, Breakey WR. Profile of the Baltimore homeless with alcohol problems. Alcohol, Health, and Research World. 1987; 11:36-41.

3. Fischer PJ. Alcohol and contemporary homelessness: An update. Paper presented at the annual meeting of the American Public Health Association, Boston, November 13-17, 1988.

4. Breakey WR. Recent empirical research on the homeless mentally ill. In Dennis D, ed. Research methodologies concerning homeless persons with serious mental illness and/or substance disorders. Proceedings of a two-day conference sponsored by the Alcohol, Drug Abuse and Mental Health Administration, July 13, 1987.

5. Schutt R, Garrett, G. Social background, residential experience, and health problems of the homeless. Psychosocial Rehab J. 1988; 12:67-70.

6. Breakey WR, Fischer PJ, Kramer M, Nestadt G, Romanoski AJ, Ross A, Royall RM, Stine OC. Health and Mental health problems of homeless men and women in Baltimore. JAMA. 1989; 262:1352-1357.

7. Schutt R, Garrett GR. The homeless alcoholic: Past and present. In Robertson M, Greenblatt M, eds. Homelessness: The national perspective. New York: Plenum, 1989.

8. Ropers RH, Boyer R. Homelessness as a health risk. Alcohol, Health and Research World. 1987; 11:38-43.

9. Rossi PH, Wright JD, Fisher GA, Willis G. The urban homeless: Estimating composition and size. Science. 1987; 235:1336-1341.

10.Ridgley MS, Goldman HH, Willenbring M. Barriers to the care of persons with dual diagnosis: Organizational and financing issues. Schiz Bull.1990; 16:123-132.

11. Kirby MW, Braucht GN. Intensive case management for homeless people with alcohol and other drug problems. Alcoholism Treatment Quarterly. 1993; 10:187-200.

12. Ridgely MS, Willenbring M. Application of case management to drug abuse treatment: Overview of models and research issues. Bethesda, MD: National Institute on Drug Abuse, 1992.

13. Levine IS, Fleming M. Human resources development: Issues in case management. Rockville, MD: National Institute of Mental Health, 1985.

14. Rog DJ, Andranovich GD, Rosenblum S. Intensive case management for individuals who are homeless and mentally ill (Vols. I, II, and III). Rockville, MD: National Institute of Mental Health, 1987.

15. Rog DJ. Engaging homeless persons with mental illness into treatment. Alexandria, VA: National Mental Health Association, 1988.

16. Intagliata J, Willer B, Egri G. The role of the family in delivering case management services. In Harris M, Bachrach LL, eds. New Directions for Mental Health Services: Clinical Case Management (No. 40). San Francisco: Jossey-Bass, 1988.

17. Robinson GK, Bergman GT. Choices in case management: Review of current knowledge and practice for mental health programs. Washington, DC: Policy Resources, Inc., 1989.

18. Joint Commission on Accreditation of Hospitals. Principles for accreditation of community mental health service programs. Chicago: Author,1979.

19. Willenbring ML, Ridgely MS, Stinchfield R, Rose M. Application of case management in alcohol and drug dependence: Matching techniques and populations. Washington, D.C., National Institute on Alcohol Abuse and Alcoholism, 1990.

20. Braucht GN, Reichardt CS. A computerized approach to trickle-process, random assignment. Evaluation Review. 1993; 17:79-90.

An Experimental Evaluation
of Residential
and Nonresidential Treatment
for Dually Diagnosed Homeless Adults

M. Audrey Burnam, PhD
Sally C. Morton, PhD
Elizabeth A. McGlynn, PhD
Laura P. Petersen, MS
Brian M. Stecher, PhD
Charles Hayes, BA
Jerome V. Vaccaro, MD

SUMMARY. Homeless adults with both a serious mental illness and substance dependence (N = 276) were randomly assigned to: (1) a social model residential program providing integrated mental health and substance abuse treatment; (2) a community-based nonresidential program using the same social model approach; or (3) a control

M. Audrey Burnam, Sally C. Morton, Elizabeth A. McGlynn, Laura P. Petersen, and Brian M. Stecher are affiliated with RAND, Santa Monica, CA.

Charles Hayes is affiliated with Social Model Recovery Systems, Los Angeles, CA.

Jerome V. Vaccaro is affiliated with the Department of Psychiatry, University of California, Los Angeles, Los Angeles, CA.

Address correspondence to M. Audrey Burnam, PhD, RAND, 1700 Main Street, P.O. Box 2138, Santa Monica, CA 90407-2138.

This research demonstration was funded by the National Institute on Alcohol Abuse and Alcoholism, as part of a multi-site cooperative agreement (#U01AA08821).

[Haworth co-indexing entry note]: "An Experimental Evaluation of Residential and Nonresidential Treatment for Dually Diagnosed Homeless Adults." Burnam, M. Audrey, et al. Co-published simultaneously in the *Journal of Addictive Diseases* (The Haworth Medical Press, an imprint of The Haworth Press, Inc.) Vol. 14, No. 4, 1995, pp. 111-134; and: *The Effectiveness of Social Interventions for Homeless Substance Abusers* (ed: Gerald J. Stahler) The Haworth Medical Press, an imprint of The Haworth Press, Inc., 1995, pp. 111-134. Single or multiple copies of this article are available from The Haworth Document Delivery Service [1-800-342-9678; 9:00 a.m. - 5:00 p.m. (EST)].

group receiving no intervention but free to access other community services. Interventions were designed to provide 3 months of intensive treatment, followed by 3 months of nonresidential maintenance. Subjects completed baseline interviews prior to randomization and reinterviews 3, 6, and 9 months later. Results showed that, while substance use, mental health, and housing outcomes improved from baseline, subjects assigned to treatment conditions differed little from control subjects. Examination of the relationship between length of treatment exposure and outcomes suggested that residential treatment had positive effects on outcomes at 3 months, but that these effects were eroded by 6 months. *[Article copies available from The Haworth Document Delivery Service: 1-800-342-9678.]*

INTRODUCTION

Following the movement in the 1960s and '70s to deinstitutionalize seriously mentally ill patients from long-term state hospital care, and in concert with the growth of the homeless population in the '80s and '90s, a new population of dually diagnosed individuals–those with both serious mental illness and substance dependence–has increasingly concerned providers in both mental health and substance abuse treatment settings. The literature indicates that these dually diagnosed individuals are at high risk of becoming homeless or relying on marginal housing arrangements.[1-6] Indeed, studies of homeless populations suggest that about 1 in 5 homeless adults have dual diagnoses.[7-10]

This new population poses difficult challenges for already strained public treatment and social welfare systems. Public mental health and substance abuse treatment have historically been delivered through separate funding streams and institutional settings, and the dually diagnosed present a clinical picture that exceeds the expertise and signals a poor prognosis in either of these separate systems.[3,8,11-14] While coordinating care across the two systems is theoretically possible, in practice differing treatment philosophies and barriers to clients presented by fragmented care have deterred the development of viable linkages between systems to better serve the needs of the dually diagnosed.[13,15] Treatment success for many dually diagnosed individuals may also be impeded by overarching needs for basic necessities such as stable housing, food, and clothing.

Such gaps in care for the dually diagnosed have stimulated the development of a number of pilot and demonstration treatment programs over the past several years. These have in common an integrated approach for treating the dually diagnosed that combines elements of traditional mental health care and substance abuse rehabilitation.[12,16-22] While these programs vary in their conceptual orientations, settings, service components, and intensity, most attempt to strike a balance between the typically nurturant and supportive approaches characterizing community-based treatment for the seriously mentally ill, and the more demanding and confrontational approach characterizing substance abuse therapeutic communities. Drug-free goals are modified to encourage appropriate use of psychotherapeutic medications. The few programs described in the literature that include a focus on persons who are both dually diagnosed and homeless have also emphasized the importance of assertive case management to assist clients in obtaining housing, income assistance, primary health care, and other needed social or educational services.

Although these emerging models of integrated treatment for dually diagnosed individuals are promising, the evaluation of such interventions to date has been greatly limited by small sample sizes, serious sample attrition, limited follow-up periods, and narrowly defined outcomes. For example, studies by Kofoed, Kania, Walsh, et al.,[16] Hellerstein and Meehan,[17] Ries and Ellingson,[23] Drake, McHugo, and Noordsy,[22] and Hoffman, DiRito, and McGill[20] all presented outcomes of treatment for dually diagnosed samples using post-assessment only designs, and none had sample sizes greater than 32. The most rigorous test of a treatment program for the dually diagnosed to date has recently been reported by Blankertz and Cnaan[21] who studied 84 subjects using a quasi-experimental design in which two treatment programs for the dually diagnosed were compared. The main outcomes that have been examined in these studies are retention in the program[16,17,21] or abstinence rates during or shortly following the treatment.[20,22] No studies in the literature to date have included an experimental design that randomizes subjects to conditions.

This report presents treatment outcome results of a research demonstration project focusing on dually diagnosed and homeless adults. The demonstration interventions were based on a social model recovery approach which combined elements of substance abuse recovery and mental illness management. The goal of this social model approach is to assist clients in developing an independent life in the community through abstinence from alcohol and street drugs and by enhancing their social and vocational abilities. The program philosophy is that this goal is best achieved in small, structured, therapeutic environments in which clients learn by interaction with one another, with staff, and with the surrounding community. Principles of this philosophy are that: (1) abstinence is prerequisite for effective program participation; (2) a program environment that is designed and maintained to dignify both clients and staff is an essential aspect of the treatment process; (3) a structured schedule of activities is needed to develop new behavior patterns; (4) a well-trained staff should provide comprehensive therapeutic services; (5) a strong, long-term case management effort is essential; (6) participation in self-help groups is an essential and ongoing aspect of recovery; and (7) each client should be respected and valued as someone with an important contribution to make to the community and society as a whole.

DEMONSTRATION INTERVENTIONS

To evaluate this intervention approach, we studied 276 homeless and dually diagnosed individuals who were randomly assigned to one of three conditions; a social model residential treatment program; a nonresidential program using the same social model approach; and a control group.

The residential treatment program was in existence prior to the initiation of the research demonstration. As part of this demonstration, treatment slots were made available to research participants without the usual 2- to 3-month waiting period that had effectively served as a barrier to homeless persons. The nonresidential program was newly implemented as part of the demonstration, and was modeled after the residential program, so that the programs operated under the same philosophy and were designed to have many common service elements. Common activities included: (1) curriculum-based groups focused on substance abuse and mental health education and rehabilitation; (2) 12-step programs including participation in community-based AA or NA meetings; (3) process-oriented groups to facilitate discussion of issues of importance to the clients; (4) individual counseling and case-management; (5) psychiatric consultation and ongoing medications management; and (6) general community activities including doing chores, helping with meal preparation, participating in sports and recreational activities, and personal time.

While the residential program was by definition a 24 hour, 7 day per week program, the nonresidential program operated in the afternoon and evening (1:00 pm to 9:00 pm) five days a week. Differences between the programs in the schedule of activities, emphasis on case management, expectations, and program rules were necessary to adapt the residential model to a nonresidential setting. For example, abstinence from drugs or alcohol was a requirement for remaining in the residential community and a single infraction confirmed with drug testing resulted in expulsion from the program. In the nonresidential setting, clients were not allowed to attend the program on any day that they were discernibly intoxicated on alcohol or drugs, but staff continued to work with these clients to engage them in the program and encourage their sobriety, irrespective of number of relapses. In addition, nonresidential clients received much more case management assistance from program staff than did residential clients, given their often pressing needs for shelter, meals, transportation, and income assistance.

Both interventions were designed to consist of a 3-month intensive phase. Successful completion of this first phase was followed by another period of 3 months during which both residential and nonresidential graduates were encouraged to continue to participate in program activities in the nonresidential setting. After the second three-month period (Phase 2), those who wished could continue to engage in program activities of their choosing. Upon completion of Phase 1, clients were invited to reside in a lightly supervised sober-living residence sponsored by the program and operated along an Oxford House model. Residents of the sober-living houses could remain as long as they wished as long as they were able to pay their share of the rent, remain sober, and get along reasonably well with other residents. Those who preferred other living arrangements were assisted in locating permanent housing. Further descriptions of the intervention can be found in McGlynn et al.[24] and Stecher et al.[25]

Those who were assigned to the control group received no special intervention, but were free to access other available community services (such as homeless shelters, a mental health clinic, a day socialization center, and AA groups). While both a public mental health clinic and a nonprofit substance abuse treatment facility serving homeless individuals were located in the community, clients who were dually diagnosed were known to be shunned by these programs.

RESEARCH METHODS

Community Setting and Research Participants

The study focused on homeless persons in the Westside area of Los Angeles County, a predominantly residential urban area that includes the two beach communities of Santa Monica and Venice, and contains a large concentration of homeless persons. While several agencies provide food, shelter and a variety of social services to homeless persons in this community, the cost of housing is generally high, access to moderately priced housing is intensely competitive, and there is substantial community resistance to the development of facilities that serve the homeless. As a result, transitional and low-income housing is very scarce, and emergency shelter facilities are able to house only about one quarter of the homeless (about 15% of men and 45% of women) on any given night.[26] Prior to this research demonstration, there were no programs on the Westside that were specifically designed to address the problems and needs of homeless and dually diagnosed individuals.

Participants were recruited from existing community agencies serving the homeless, including shelters, day centers, a substance abuse program, and a mental health clinic. Potential participants were either individually referred from an agency to research staff, or research staff visited agencies and directly approached their clients. Those who agreed to be interviewed by research staff participated in a brief screening interview which established whether or not participants met criteria for homelessness (either literally homeless or lived in two or more dependent housing situations in the past 6 months), and screened for symptoms of serious mental illness and a history of problems with alcohol or drugs. Those who met criteria at this stage were asked to participate in a structured diagnostic interview administered by nonclinician interviewers (the Diagnostic Interview Schedule, Version III-R) to confirm diagnoses. Those meeting lifetime DSM III-R criteria for schizophrenia or major affective disorder, and also criteria for substance dependence (with some substance abuse or dependence problems in the past year) were eligible for the study. Of those who participated in the initial screening interview (N = 1112), 64% met initial eligibility criteria. Among screener eligibles (N = 717), 81% completed the diagnostic interview. Of those completing the diagnostic interview (N = 583), 83% (N = 484) were fully eligible for study participation.

Among persons determined to be eligible, 57% (N = 276) agreed to participate in the study and be randomly assigned to conditions. After completing baseline interviews, these subjects were randomly assigned to nonresidential treatment (N = 144), residential treatment (N = 67), or the control group (N = 65). Probability of assignment to the nonresidential group was set at twice that of the other groups because we expected a higher degree of variability in exposure to treatment for those assigned to this intervention, and would therefore need a relatively larger sample size to detect a treatment effect. Random assignment was made within two blocking variables, gender and primary type of mental disorder (schizophrenia versus affective). Study participants were asked to complete follow-up interviews at 3 months, 6 months, and 9 months following their baseline interviews. The 3-month interview occurred around the time of completing treatment Phase 1 (among those who stayed in treatment). Participants were sought for follow-up interviews during a 2-month window of time spanning their scheduled follow-up date whether or not they were in treatment. Those who were not found for one follow-up interview were again sought for subsequent interviews. Participants were paid $2 for completing the initial screening interview, and $10 for completing each of the diagnostic interview, baseline interview, and follow-up interviews. Those who called in to schedule an appointment for their follow-up interviews (using a toll-free number) were given an additional $2.

Measures

The evaluation of the treatment interventions focused on the three major outcome domains: substance use, severity of mental illness symptoms, and housing status. Questions regarding substance use asked about frequency (and in the case of alcohol, quantity) of use of different categories of drugs in the past 30 days. Four measures of substance use were constructed: (1) number of days consumed any alcohol in the past 30; (2) number of days used any illicit drugs in the past 30; (3) a quantity index reflecting 3 levels of alcohol use in the past 30 days: abstinence, low quantity consumption (less than 3 oz. absolute alcohol or 5 drinks on any day), and high quantity consumption (at least 3 oz. absolute alcohol or 5 drinks on at least one day), based on a measure developed by Pollich and colleagues;[27] and (4) a drug use index weighting frequency of use by the severity of the drug used, as suggested by Phin,[28] and modified by Bray and colleagues.[29] Mental illness symptom questions referred to the past 7 days, and covered dimensions of depression, anxiety, psychoticism, anger/hostility, taken from the SCL-90,[30-32] with mania and self-esteem scales included from the Psychiatric Epidemiologic Research Interview (PERI).[33] Internal reliability of each of these scales was high (Cronbach's alphas ranged from .60 for mania to .82 for self-esteem). The depression and anxiety scales were combined into one because of lack of discriminant validity between the separate scales, and the resulting scales adequately reflect discrete dimensions, with interscale correlations ranging from 0 to .5. To assess recent housing and homelessness patterns, the interview asked subjects to provide a history of their living arrangements over the past 60 days, which were classified into the following categories: on the streets (including abandoned buildings, parked cars, bus depots, parks); independent housing (own house, apartment, room, boarding house, group home); and dependent housing (emergency shelters, health and correctional facilities, doubled up with family or friends). The housing status measures we used in analyses of outcomes were the percentage of nights in the past 60 that respondents spent on streets and the percentage of nights spent in independent housing, with the percentage of nights spent in dependent housing as the omitted category.

Prognostic and history variables measured at baseline that were considered as covariates in analyses of outcomes included demographic characteristics (gender, age, race, marital status, veteran status, educational level), primary thought versus mood disorder, number of symptoms of alcohol dependence in the past year, number of symptoms of drug disorder in the past year, presence of antisocial personality, number of years homeless, satisfaction with physical health, prior hospitalization for psychiatric problems, and prior substance abuse treatment. In addition, other history variables were considered as covariates for specific outcome domains. For substance use outcomes, we examined the number of years subjects had regularly used alcohol to the point of getting high or drunk, number of years they had used any other drugs regularly, ever had alcohol DTs, ever overdosed on drugs (all taken from The Addiction Severity Index,[34] and the Alcohol Dependence Scale[35]). For housing outcomes, we included age at which subjects first became homeless. For mental health symptom outcomes, we considered age of first major symptom of schizophrenia or affective disorder, and the presence of episodes of schizophrenia, major depression, and mania in the past year.

The study also assessed out-of-program treatment received by both the experimental treatment and control groups at baseline and in each follow-up period. Measures used in analyses to control for out-of-program treatment exposure included: (1) the log of days of attendance at AA (12-step) meetings in the past 30 days (not counted if the client was active in the experimental treatment interventions during the past month, since attendance at AA meetings was a component of the intervention); (2) any use of prescribed psychotherapeutic medications in the past 30 days; (3) any inpatient or outpatient treatment for a mental health problem in the past 30 days; and (4) any formal treatment (residential or nonresidential) for a substance abuse problem in the past 30 days.

Analysis

Two sets of analyses were conducted to examine the effects of treatment on outcomes, testing whether: (1) outcomes differ across subjects assigned to nonresidential vs. residential treatment groups; and (2) outcomes differ between those assigned to treatment vs. control groups (with residential and nonresidential conditions combined). General linear regression models were used to examine treatment effects, with the difference score between baseline and follow-up outcome measures constituting the dependent variable, and treatment assignment as the independent variable. Because we did not adjust the variances for our stratified random design effect that resulted from blocking prior to randomization, our regression coefficient tests are conservative. Separate analyses were performed for each baseline to follow-up difference score (i.e., baseline to 3 months, baseline to 6 months, baseline to 9 months) and for each of the 11 outcome measures. Difference scores were constructed so that, across all outcome measures, a positive score indicated improvement in functioning, while a negative score indicated decline in functioning. Unadjusted regression models included only treatment assignment as a predictor of outcome difference scores, while adjusted regression models included both treatment assignment and relevant baseline covariates as predictors. Given our relatively small sample size, a parsimonious covariate selection procedure was required to deal with the large number of potential covariates. Relevant covariates to include in the models were thus selected using backwards stepwise linear regression to identify those significantly associated with the outcome domain irrespective of group assignment. The stepwise selection procedure was used within each outcome domain (such as substance use), and covariates which were consistently significant for outcomes within this domain were selected. The set of selected covariates was therefore identical for each outcome within a domain but differed across domains.

A final set of regression analyses tested whether level of treatment exposure predicted outcomes at each of the follow-up periods, with exposure measured as the log number of days subjects participated in the treatment program. Because exposure to treatment was self-selected, each of these models included baseline covariates to control as much as possible for self-selection biases. Indicators of out-of-program exposure to substance use and mental health services were then added to the models to control for potential contamination of the treatment versus control group comparisons.

RESULTS

Study Sample and Attrition

The characteristics of the 276 persons who completed a baseline interview and were randomly assigned to one of the three study conditions are shown in Table 1. The large majority were unmarried males in their 30s and 40s with at least a high school degree. The sample was nearly equal in the distribution of primary schizophrenia versus major affective disorder. Both drug and alcohol dependence were highly prevalent, with many individuals reporting problems across multiple substances. In the past month, 53% of the sample had used cocaine, 47% used marijuana, 24% used sedatives, 9% used opiates, 8% used amphetamines, 6% used hallucinogens, and 3% used barbiturates and inhalants. While the three study groups were closely comparable at baseline in most characteristics that

TABLE 1. Characteristics of Sample by Treatment Group Assignment.

	Nonresidential Treatment	Residential Treatment	Controls	Total
	(N = 144)	(N = 67)	(N = 65)	(N = 276)
% Male	83	81	89	84
Mean Age (in years)	37	36	37	37
Race				
% White	56	57	65	58
% Black	30	31	21	28
% Other	14	12	14	14
Marital Status**				
% Currently married	5	15	0	6
% Previously married	47	46	40	45
% Never married	48	39	60	49
% Veteran	34	33	40	35
Education				
% < High School	29	27	25	28
% High School	29	39	41	34
% Some College	42	34	34	38
Mean Years Homeless	4.9	3.7	5.1	4.7
Mean no. of nights slept on street of past 60	49	49	51	49
Mental Disorder				
% Schizophrenia only	7	6	8	7
% Major affective only	56	60	48	55
% Both	37	34	44	38
Alcohol Disorder in past year	79	76	80	79
Mean no. symptoms	3.8	3.4	3.8	3.7
Drug Disorder in past year	74	72	69	72
Mean no. symptoms	3.9	4.2	3.5	3.9

**Significant difference among groups at $p < .01$

were examined, there was a significant difference across groups in their marital status. We note that only this 1 significant difference was found among 15 variables tested that included 4 not shown in Table 1: presence of antisocial personality, satisfaction with physical health status, prior hospitalizations for psychiatric problems, and prior treatment for substance abuse problems. This high degree of similarity across groups provides assurance that randomization procedures were appropriately implemented and resulted in comparable groups.

Rates of completed follow-up interviews among the 276 study participants were 79% for the 3-month follow-up, 76% for the 6-month follow-up, 70% for the 9-month follow-up, and 58% completed all three follow-ups. Follow-up completion rates were not different across the three treatment conditions, except at the 9-month follow-up, where the completion rate among those assigned to the control group (57%) was significantly lower than among those assigned to nonresidential treatment (76%).

While this is a relatively low level of attrition for a longitudinal study of homeless persons, we were concerned that it had the potential to introduce bias into the findings, if factors associated with study attrition differed across groups. To determine whether differential attrition was a concern, we tested whether the three treatment groups remained comparable at each of the follow-up periods with respect to the fifteen baseline variables described above. These analyses showed that the three study groups differed in satisfaction with physical health status at the three-month follow-up; the residential and nonresidential groups differed in marital status at six months; and the control group differed from both the residential and nonresidential groups in marital status at nine months. Considering that multiple tests were conducted, this relatively small number of significant results suggests that the study groups were largely comparable at each of the follow-up timepoints.

Nonresidential and Residential Treatment Outcomes

No significant differences were found between nonresidential and residential treatment groups at any of the three follow-up periods for any of the outcomes examined, with the exception of time spent in independent housing at the 3-month follow-up (see Table 2). Those assigned to nonresidential treatment were more likely to have increased the amount of time they spent in independent housing at 3 months following baseline, relative to those in residential treatment. This finding is expected because the 3-month follow-up was scheduled immediately after the first phase of treatment completion, and subjects in residential treatment were by definition not independently housed. While Table 2 provides adjusted mean differ-

TABLE 2. Adjusted differences in substance use, mental health, and housing patterns over time by residential versus nonresidential treatment assignment.

| Group Assignment | Mean at Baseline† | | Mean differences from Baseline to Follow-up Assessment†† | | | | | |
| | | | 3-Month Follow-up | | 6-Month Follow-up | | 9-Month Follow-up | |
	Nonresidential (N = 144)	Residential (N = 67)	Nonresidential (N = 114)	Residential (N = 57)	Nonresidential (N = 114)	Residential (N = 49)	Nonresidential (N = 110)	Residential (N = 45)
Substance Use in Past 30 days								
Days used alcohol	11.4	11.5	4.5	6.5	3.8	3.8	5.6	4.6
Level alcohol use	1.4	1.5	0.4	0.7	0.3	0.4	0.4	0.3
Days used drugs	9.8	8.3	3.1	5.2	2.6	1.9	3.9	3.4
Severity drug use	4.2	3.7	1.2	1.6	0.8	0.8	1.9	1.5
Current Mental Health Symptoms								
Depression and anxiety	52	55	7.5	8.6	6.2	10.0	9.5	13.8
Psychotic symptoms	25	25	3.0	0.4	3.4	6.1	5.6	4.0
Anger and hostility	27	28	-0.6	-0.9	-2.9	2.4	-0.8	-1.4
Mania	32	37	-0.5	3.7	0.0	0.6	0.5	2.6
Self esteem	47	50	8.5	4.5	8.0	9.6	5.6	4.0
Housing Status in Past 60 days								
% time on streets	52	48	20	25	27	27	21	19
% time in independent housing	18	16	15*	-1	19	33	18	14

† Range for "days used alcohol" and "days used drugs" was 0 to 30 days. "Level alcohol use" ranged from 0 (none) to heavy (2) while "severity drug use" was scored from 0 to 75. Measures of mental health symptoms and housing status all ranged from 0 to 100.

†† Underlined differences are significantly different from zero (no change from baseline) at p < .05. Positive numbers indicate improvement in outcome from baseline to follow-up (less substance use, better mental health, less time homeless on streets, more time independently housed); while negative numbers indicate poorer outcome from baseline to follow-up.

*Difference between residential and nonresidential treatment group is significant at p < .05.

ences in scores between baseline and follow-up measures, controlling for relevant baseline covariates, results were similar for analyses of unadjusted means. Table 2 also shows that both nonresidential and residential treatment groups reported significant improvement in many outcomes from baseline to follow-up assessments, especially for measures of substance use, symptoms of depression/anxiety, self-esteem, and indicators of housing status. No improvement was evidenced in measures of psychotic symptoms, mania, or anger/hostility.

We then combined residential and nonresidential treatment assignment groups and compared the outcomes of those assigned to treatment to those assigned to the no-treatment control group. In spite of significant improvements between baseline and follow-up assessments across most outcome measures in the treatment groups, there were few significant differences between the treatment and control groups in outcomes (see Table 3). The only outcome measure for which treatment groups displayed a significantly greater improvement than the control group was days of alcohol use at the 3-month follow-up. For many outcomes, the control group, like the treatment groups, showed improvements from baseline to follow-up assessments. Unadjusted mean comparisons gave similar results to the adjusted mean comparisons shown here.

Exposure to Treatment and Its Relationship to Outcomes

Although both the nonresidential and residential programs made efforts to engage all subjects assigned to treatment, 40% of those assigned to either program never attended, with no difference in nonattendance rates between the nonresidential and residential programs. Among those who attended, retention was higher in the residential than the nonresidential program. In the residential program, 49% of those assigned stayed in the program for at least two weeks, and 24% successfully completed Phase 1. In the nonresidential program, only 36% of those assigned attended as much as 2 weeks of the program over the study period (10 program days), and only 8% successfully completed Phase 1.

Results of analyses examining changes in outcomes between baseline and follow-up as a function of log days of residential and nonresidential program exposure, controlling for treatment group assignment and relevant baseline covariates, are shown in Table 4. Significant treatment exposure effects were found for residential treatment across substance use and housing outcomes at the 3-month follow-up, indicating that longer retention in residential treatment was associated with better outcomes. However, these positive effects of residential treatment exposure found at 3 months were not maintained at the 6- and 9-month follow-ups, with the exception of

TABLE 3. Adjusted difference in substance use, mental health symptoms, and housing patterns over time by treatment versus control group assignment.

Group Assignment	Mean at Baseline[†]		Mean differences from Baseline to Follow-up Assessment[††]					
			3-Month Follow-up		6-Month Follow-up		9-Month Follow-up	
	Treatment (N=211)	Control (N=65)	Treatment (N=171)	Control (N=47)	Treatment (N=163)	Control (N=48)	Treatment (N=155)	Control (N=37)
Substance Use in Past 30 days								
Days used alcohol	11.4	12.3	5.2 **	0.6	3.6	3.8	5.3	5.4
Level alcohol use	1.5	1.6	0.5	0.2	0.3	0.5	0.4	0.6
Days used drugs	9.3	4.5	3.8	1.4	2.4	3.8	3.8	3.9
Severity drug use	4.1	4.5	1.3	0.7	0.8 *	2.2	1.8	2.5
Current Mental Health Symptoms								
Depression and anxiety	53	53	7.9	7.5	7.3	13.4	10.8	15.5
Psychotic symptoms	25	27	2.1	3.9	4.2	4.9	5.2	7.0
Anger and hostility	27	27	-0.1	-7.8	-1.3	2.8	-1.0	2.5
Mania	34	32	0.9	0.2	0.2	2.5	1.1	6.2
Self esteem	49	47	7.2	4.4	8.5	7.1	6.2	2.8
Housing Status in Past 60 days								
% time on streets	51	53	22	22	27	22	21	26
% time in independent housing	17	14	10	11	23	14	17	29

[†] Range for "days used alcohol" and "days used drugs" was 0 to 30 days. "Level alcohol use" ranged from 0 (none) to heavy (2) while "severity drug use" was scored from 0 to 75. Measures of mental health symptoms and housing status all ranged from 0 to 100.
[††] Underlined differences are significantly different from zero (no change from baseline) at p < .05. Positive numbers indicate improvement in outcome from baseline to follow-up (less substance use, better mental health, less time homeless on streets, more time independently housed); while negative numbers indicate poorer outcome from baseline to follow-up.
*Difference between treatment and control group is significant at p < .05.
**Difference between treatment and control group is significant at p < .01.

124

TABLE 4. Relationship of treatment exposure to changes in substance use, mental health, and housing patterns.

	Regression Coefficients for Significant Effects of Treatment Exposure on Differences in Outcomes Between Baseline and Follow-up Assessments[t]					
	3-month Follow-up		6-month Follow-up		9-month Follow-up	
	Non-res. days	Res. days	Non-res. days	Res. days	Non-res. days	Res. days
Substance Use in Past 30 Days						
Days used alcohol		1.73	1.49			
Level alcohol use		0.16				
Days used drugs		1.70				
Severity drug use						
Current Mental Health Symptoms						
Depression and anxiety						
Psychotic symptoms						
Anger and hostility						
Mania						
Self-esteem						
Housing Status in Past 60 days						
% time on streets		0.03				
% time in independent housing				0.08		

[t] Regression coefficients are shown for treatment exposure effects that were significant predictors of outcomes, controlling for treatment assignment and baseline covariates. All other treatment exposure coefficients were nonsignificant.

improvements in independent housing at 6 months. Days of nonresidential treatment participation had less discernible effect on outcomes, showing only one significant association with days of alcohol use at 6 months, and no significant association with outcomes at 3 or 9 months.

When indicators of out-of-program treatment were added to these regression models to control for possible contamination of the experimental treatment effect through use of other substance abuse and mental health related services (see Table 5), further significant effects of exposure to nonresidential and residential treatment emerged. Exposure to nonresidential treatment, in addition to predicting improved substance use outcomes at 6 months, was also associated with improvements in depression/anxiety

TABLE 5. Relationship of Treatment Exposure and Out-of-Program Treatment to Changes in Substance Use, Mental Health, and Housing Patterns.

	Regression Coefficients for Significant Treatment Exposure and Out-of-Program Treatment on Differences in Outcomes Between Baseline and Follow-Up Assessments[†]																	
	3-month Follow-Up						6-month Follow-Up						9-month Follow-Up					
	Study Intervention		Out-of-Program Treatment[*]				Study Intervention		Out-of-Program Treatment[*]				Study Intervention		Out-of-Program Treatment[*]			
	Non-res. days	Res. days	AA	Meds	MH TX	SA TX	Non-res. days	Res. days	AA	Meds	MH TX	SA TX	Non-res. days	Res. days	AA	Meds	MH TX	SA TX
Substance Use in Past 30 days																		
Days used alcohol	1.97	1.68							2.14						2.22		5.59	
Level alcohol use			0.17				0.13		0.17									
Days used drugs	1.96	1.60													1.76		4.24	
Severity drug use															0.62			
Current Mental Health Symptoms																		
Depression and anxiety	3.33	4.09	3.52															
Psychotic symptoms				−13.0	8.09	−11.4												

126

Anger and hostility	4.01	5.20	
Mania			
Self-esteem	3.77	−10.3	−8.22
Housing Status in Past 60 days			
% time on streets	0.08		
% time in independent housing			

¹Regression coefficients are shown for treatment exposure effects that were predictors of outcomes, controlling for treatment assignment and baseline covariates. All other treatment exposure coefficients were nonsignificant.
"AA" is log of days attended 12-step meetings in past 30, "Meds" is any use of prescribed psychotherapeutic medications in past 30 days, "MH TX" is any inpatient or outpatient mental health treatment in the past 30 days, "SA TX" is any formal treatment (residential or non-residential) for a substance problem in the past 30 days.

at 3 months. Exposure to residential treatment, in addition to having positive effects on substance use and housing outcomes at 3 months, was also associated with improvements in two measures of mental health status at 3 months (depression/anxiety, anger/hostility). The effect of nonresidential treatment on housing status at 6 months, however, was reduced to nonsignificance.

These analyses also showed that indicators of out-of-program treatment were sometimes significantly associated with outcomes. Of particular interest is the association of attendance at AA meetings with improvements in substance use outcomes at all three follow-up periods, and also with improvements in mental health symptoms (depression/anxiety, anger/hostility, and self-esteem) at the 3-month follow-up. Use of psychotherapeutic medications was generally not associated with outcomes, except for a negative association with psychotic symptoms at 3 months, perhaps reflecting a reverse causal association (that is, those with increasing levels of psychotic symptoms being more likely to get and use medications). Out-of-program mental health treatment was associated with some positive outcomes (improvements in psychotic symptoms at 3 months and substance use at 9 months), but was also related to lower self-esteem at 3 and 9 months. Out-of-program substance abuse treatment had no discernible association with outcomes, except for an association with increased psychotic symptoms at 3 months that is not readily interpretable.

DISCUSSION

The most rigorous test of the effectiveness of a treatment intervention is the experimental design, in which subjects are randomly assigned to treatment and control groups, and the outcomes of all persons assigned are compared between groups. Using this evaluation standard, we found little discernible effect of intensive integrated treatment on substance use, mental health, or housing outcomes among dually diagnosed and homeless adults. On only one measure, frequency of alcohol use, did the treatment groups show more improvement than the control group. And this positive effect, while significant at the end of the 3-month intensive phase of treatment, was not detectable at the 6- or 9-month follow-ups. Because our sample sizes were adequate for detecting medium-sized effects (0.5), the absence of detectable treatment effects cannot be attributed to insufficient statistical power.

Previous studies of integrated treatment interventions for dually diagnosed individuals have reported positive outcomes with much smaller sample sizes, but have not employed experimental designs, and often excluded from analysis persons who dropped out of treatment early. Both of these design weaknesses are likely to have biased results towards finding positive effects of treatment. In the case of nonexperimental pre- and post-treatment comparisons, simple regression to the mean could explain improvements from before to after treatment, particularly if subjects are selected into treatment during a period of acute problems with substance abuse and/or mental illness. Such regression to the mean could explain why, in the present study, the control as well as the treatment groups showed improvements in many outcomes from baseline to follow-up assessments. Another possible explanation for improvements in the control as well as the treatment groups is that the control group was "contaminated" by its exposure to other types of mental health, substance abuse, and homeless services. This explanation suggests that the improvements in the treatment groups from baseline to follow-up assessments are truly positive outcomes of treatment rather than regressions to a mean level of functioning, but that the control group also improved as a result of the variety of services that it received and therefore masked the differences between the treatment and control conditions. Perhaps those assigned to the control conditions were nonetheless stimulated by the research protocol to seek help for their substance abuse and mental health problems. In analyses designed to partial out the contaminating effects of use of services received outside of the experimental treatment interventions, significant treatment exposure effects were found, but these were largely restricted to a positive impact of residential treatment on substance use and mental health at the 3-month follow-up (occurring at the end of the intensive treatment period). These results suggest that residential treatment effects were real, but short-lived, and that regression to the mean may explain apparent pre-post improvements in outcomes over the longer period of evaluation.

While it is common in treatment evaluation studies to exclude from analysis subjects who drop out of treatment early, this practice can seriously bias results if, as many clinicians believe, those clients who are more likely to have poor outcomes anyway are also most likely to drop out of treatment and those who have a good prognosis most likely to stay in. For this reason, we included in our analyses all persons who agreed to be assigned to either a treatment or control group. Conceptually, one can think of this as a test of the effectiveness of the programs' "intention" to provide treatment to a targeted group of individuals. This is the most rigorous and appropriate test of treatment because it avoids biases introduced by selective treatment retention. At the same time, it raises concerns that high rates of early drop-out from both treatment programs may have diluted real treatment effects among those who had more exposure to the interventions.

When we analyzed the relationship of days of treatment exposure to outcomes, a consistent effect of residential treatment on improved outcomes at 3 months did, in fact, emerge. Because we had comprehensively assessed variables that might be expected to predict outcomes at baseline, and included these as covariates in our models, we can cautiously assert that exposure to a 3-month intensive social model residential treatment intervention improved outcomes over what would have been expected in this dually diagnosed and homeless population, but only for a short period of time.

One issue that merits special attention with this population is the limited extent to which newly emerging programs specifically designed for the dually diagnosed appear to have been successful in engaging them in sustained treatment efforts. Among studies reporting any information about treatment drop-outs, most report high rates of early program attrition: 66% dropped out of a once-a-week VA outpatient group within 2 months in Kofoed and colleagues' pilot study;[16] five out of ten clients dropped out of another weekly outpatient group within 1 year as reported by Hellerstein and Meehan;[17] Blankertz and Cnaan[21] give drop-out rates of 43% and 106% among homeless dually diagnosed clients within the first 2 months of a structured residence program and modified therapeutic community, respectively. Drop-out rates in the present demonstration were also high. Among those who attended at least once, drop-out rates in the first two weeks were 18% and 40% in the residential and nonresidential groups, respectively. If those who agreed to participate in the demonstration but never entered treatment are included, these early drop-out rates increase to 51% and 64%. While some treatment attrition is to be expected, particularly for programs demanding sobriety of substance abusers, the dually diagnosed seem particularly difficult to engage in treatment even when it is specially targeted to their comorbid disorders.

In hindsight, we speculate that engagement and retention of this population could have been improved by restructuring the intervention in two ways. First, an extended and low-demand first phase of entry into the program may have boosted participation. It is our impression that some individuals who were not quite "ready" to commit themselves to treatment at the time they entered the demonstration would over time have become involved given a more flexible and low-demand option for engaging. This idea has been articulated by others[10,36] as a model in which clients progress, or regress if necessary, through different phases of treatment, with engagement and persuasion as the first phases (for example, through mental health treatment settings where abstinence is a goal but not a requirement), followed by more active treatment and relapse prevention (with higher expectations for abstinence and a focus on skills to maintain abstinence).

Second, we think that our treatment approach underestimated the primacy of housing and income needs in this population, and the difficulties involved in assisting clients with such needs even with intensive case management. This was particularly a problem for clients in the nonresidential program, who usually required immediate efforts to secure temporary shelter and apply for disability and/or welfare income assistance. Because housing of any type was difficult to access in this community (including emergency or transitional housing as well as permanent housing), program staff were often frustrated in their efforts. We believe that low-demand but highly supervised transitional housing linked to the nonresidential program would have increased its effectiveness in engaging and retaining clients. Expanded affordable permanent housing options for both residential and nonresidential clients upon completion of the initial intensive phase of treatment might have facilitated continued treatment involvement and gains in sobriety. Although a project-sponsored sober-living house and apartments were available, the financial feasibility of this option was dependent upon all residents contributing their share to the monthly rent, and upon fully occupied dwellings (2 residents per bedroom). The sober living homes failed to attract and maintain many treatment graduates because of their expense (only those who had qualified for and received SSI could afford the rent), the inability of some clients to live cooperatively and in close quarters with others, and the requirement that residents remain abstinent. In addition to the universal need, in our target population, for very low- or no-cost housing options, a range of housing environments in addition to sober-living homes such as single apartments, supervised community support residences or half-way houses, and moderately "wet" transitional housing would have better served the range of residential needs that existed.

Our experience has also led us to question the appropriateness of applying relatively short-term treatment models to the joint problems of serious mental illness and substance dependence. Serious mental illness is by definition the presence of a persistent and often lifelong disorder characterized by acute exacerbations and serious functional impairment. The natural course of substance addiction is also typically prolonged or chronic, characterized by multiple episodes of remittance and relapse among treated populations. Given this reality, it is perhaps not surprising that a relatively short-term intervention would have little detectable and lasting impact. What may be needed to stabilize and maximize the functioning of dually diagnosed individuals is a model of care that is very long-term and continuous, such as that described by Drake, McHugo, and Noordsy[22] who report high rates of abstinence among 18 individuals who were treated continuously in an integrated dual diagnosis program over a period of four years. In this regard, an interesting finding from our study is that those subjects who attended AA meetings, beyond participation in the experimental treatment interventions, had better substance use outcomes over the course of the 9-month evaluation. This finding must be interpreted cautiously because it is possible to explain as an individual selection effect (that is, individuals who have better outcomes are more likely to attend AA meetings) and cannot conclusively be attributed to the efficacy of AA involvement. Nonetheless AA groups do have the advantage of providing a continuously available–even lifelong–source of support for this population, unlike formal treatment programs. While long-term support for sobriety may increase positive outcomes among the homeless dually diagnosed, we think it unlikely that any program, formal or self-help, is likely to produce long-lasting benefits unless issues of housing and income support are also resolved for this population.

REFERENCES

1. Koegel P, Burnam MA. Alcoholism among homeless adults in the inner-city of Los Angeles. Arch Gen Psychiatry 1988; 45:1011-1018.

2. Drake RE, Wallach MA, Schuyler Hoffman J. Housing instability and homelessness among aftercare patients of an urban state hospital. Hosp Comm Psychiatry 1989; 40:46-51.

3. Drake RE, Wallach MA. Substance abuse among the chronic mentally ill. Hosp Comm Psychiatry 1989; 40:1041-1046.

4. Belcher JR. On becoming homeless: A study of chronically mentally ill persons. J Comm Psychology 1989; 17:173-185.

5. Drake RE, Wallach MA, Teague GB, et al. Housing instability and homelessness among rural schizophrenic patients. Am J Psychiatry 1991; 148:330-336.

6. Caton CLM, Wyatt RJ, Felix A, et al. Follow-up of chronically homeless mentally ill men. Am J Psychiatry 1993; 150:1639-1642.

7. Koegel P, Burnam MA. Traditional and nontraditional homeless alcoholics. Alcohol Health & Research World 1987; 11:28-34.

8. Vernez G, Burnam MA, McGlynn EA, et al. Review of California's program for the homeless mentally disabled. Santa Monica, CA: RAND 1988; (RAND Report R-3631-CDMH).

9. Fischer PJ, Breakey WR. The epidemiology of alcohol, drug, and mental disorders among homeless persons. Am Psychologist 1991; 46:1115-1128.

10. Drake RE, Osher FC, Wallach MA. Homelessness and dual diagnosis. Am Psychologist 1991; 46:1149-1158.

11. Drake RE, Osher FC, Wallach MA. Alcohol use and abuse in schizophrenia: A prospective community study. J Nerv Ment Dis 1989; 177:408-414.

12. Osher FC, Kofoed LL. Treatment of patients with psychiatric and psychoactive substance abuse disorders. Hosp Comm Psychiatry 1989; 40: 1025-1030.

13. Ridgely MS, Goldman HH, Willenbring M. Barriers to the care of persons with dual diagnoses: Organizational and financing issues. Schizophrenia Bulletin 1990; 16:123-132.

14. Salloum IM, Moss HB, Daley DC. Substance abuse and schizophrenia: Impediments to optimal care. Am J Drug Alcohol Abuse 1991; 17:321-336.

15. Bachrach LL. Issues in identifying and treating the homeless mentally ill. New Directions for Mental Health Services 1987; 35:43-62.

16. Kofoed L, Kania J, Walsh T, et al. Outpatient treatment of patients with substance abuse and coexisting psychiatric disorders. Am J Psychiatry 1986; 143:867-872.

17. Hellerstein DJ, Meehan B. Outpatient group therapy for schizophrenic substance abusers. Am J Psychiatry 1987; 144:1337-1339.

18. Noordsy DL, Fox L. Group intervention techniques for people with dual disorders. Psychosocial Rehabilitation Journal 1991; 15:67-78.

19. Bartels SJ, Thomas WN. Lessons from a pilot residential treatment program for people with dual diagnoses of severe mental illness and substance use disorder. Psychosocial Rehabilitation Journal 1991; 15:19- 30.

20. Hoffman Jr. GW, DiRito DC, McGill EC. Three-month follow-up of 28 dual diagnosis inpatients. Am J Drug Alcohol Abuse 1993; 19:79-88.

21. Blankertz LE, Cnaan RA. Serving the dually diagnosed homeless: Program development and interventions. J Ment Health Admin 1993; 20:100- 111.

22. Drake RE, McHugo GJ, Noordsy DL. Treatment of alcoholism among schizophrenic outpatients: 4-year outcomes. Am J Psychiatry 1993; 150:328-329.

23. Ries RK, Ellingson T. A pilot assessment at one month of 17 dual diagnosis patients. Hosp Comm Psychiatry 1990; 41:1230-1233.

24. McGlynn EA, Boynton J, Morton SC, et al. Treatment for the dually diagnosed homeless: Program models and implementation experience. Alcoholism Treatment Quarterly 1993; 10:171-186.

25. Stecher BM, Andrews CA, McDonald L, et al. Implementation of residential and nonresidential treatment for the dually diagnosed homeless. Eval Rev 1994; 18:689-717.

26. Koegel P, Burnam MA, Morton SC. Enumerating homeless people: Alternative strategies and their consequences. Eval Rev, in press.

27. Polich JM, Armor DJ, Braiker HB. The course of alcoholism: Four years after treatment. New York: John Wiley & Sons, 1981.

28. Phin J. Nonpatient polydrug users. In Wesson DR, Carlin AS, Adams KM, et al., eds. Polydrug abuse. The results of a national collaborative study. New York: Academic Press, 1978.

29. Bray RM, Schlenger WE, Craddock SG, et al. Approaches to the assessment of drug use in the treatment outcome prospective study. Treatment Outcome Prospective Study, Research Triangle Institute, Research Triangle Park, NC, March 1982.

30. Derogatis LR, Lipman RS, Covi L. SCL-90: An outpatient psychiatric rating scale: Preliminary report. Psychopharmacology Bulletin 1973; 9:13-27.

31. Derogatis LR, Yevzeroff H, Wittelsberger B. Social class, psychological disorder, and the nature of the psychopathologic indicator. Journal of Consulting and Clinical Psychology 1975; 43:183-191.

32. Derogatis LR, Rickels K, Rock A. The SCL-90 and the MMPI: A step in the validation of a new self-report scale. Brit J Psych 1976; 128:280-289.

33. Dohrenwend BP, Shrout PE, Egri G, et al. Nonspecific psychological distress and other dimensions of psychopathology. Arch Gen Psychiatry 1980; 37: 1229-1236.

34. McLellan AT, Luborsky L, Cacciola J, et al. Guide to the addiction severity index: Background, administration, and field testing results. Washington, DC: National Institute on Drug Abuse, 1988.

35. Horn JL, Skinner HA, Wanberg K, et al. Alcohol Dependence Scale (ADS). Toronto: Addiction Research Foundation of Ontario, 1984.

36. Minkoff K. An integrated treatment model for dual diagnosis of psychosis and addiction. Hosp Comm Psychiatry 1989; 40:1031-1036.

Willingness for Treatment as a Predictor of Retention and Outcomes

Julie Reed Erickson, PhD
Sally Stevens, PhD
Patrick McKnight, MS
Aurelio Jose Figueredo, PhD

SUMMARY. Retention in drug treatment is important to successful outcomes. The purpose of this study was to test assumptions made in the development and implementation of the ASSET project. The three assumptions were that living conditions of the homeless adult drug user influence willingness for treatment; willingness relates to treatment tenure; and, conditions, willingness and time in treatment influence treatment outcomes. Data on alcohol use, drug use, employment and housing as well as motivation, readiness and suitability of treatment were collected from 494 homeless adults at baseline and at follow-up. Data were subjected to multivariate causal analysis using factor analytic structural equations modeling. Practical fit indices were acceptable. The measurement model confirmed a higher order

Julie Reed Erickson is affiliated with the College of Nursing, The University of Arizona, Tucson, AZ.

Sally Stevens is affiliated with Amity, Inc.

Patrick McKnight and Aurelio Jose Figueredo are affiliated with the Department of Psychology, The University of Arizona, Tucson, AZ.

Address correspondence to Julie Reed Erickson, College of Nursing, The University of Arizona, 1401 North Martin, Tucson, AZ 85721.

This research was supported by the National Institute on Alcohol Abuse and Alcoholism, Grant #U01 AA08788.

[Haworth co-indexing entry note]: "Willingness for Treatment as a Predictor of Retention and Outcomes." Erickson, Julie Reed, et al. Co-published simultaneously in the *Journal of Addictive Diseases* (The Haworth Medical Press, an imprint of The Haworth Press, Inc.) Vol. 14, No. 4, 1995, pp. 135-150; and: *The Effectiveness of Social Interventions for Homeless Substance Abusers* (ed: Gerald J. Stahler) The Haworth Medical Press, an imprint of The Haworth Press, Inc., 1995, pp. 135-150. Single or multiple copies of this article are available from The Haworth Document Delivery Service [1-800-342-9678; 9:00 a.m. - 5:00 p.m. (EST)].

135

construct labelled willingness encompassing motivation, readiness and suitability. The structural model demonstrated that willingness positively related to treatment tenure; willingness positively influenced change in drug use and housing; and, tenure related positively to change in housing. *[Article copies available from The Haworth Document Delivery Service: 1-800-342-9678.]*

For drug users, retention in treatment is related to successful outcomes.[1-10] In Therapeutic Communities (TCs), clients who stay longer in treatment have less drug use and lower unemployment at discharge and in posttreatment years than do clients with shorter tenures.[11-15] Condelli and De Leon [10] report that retention rates in TCs are lower than methadone maintenance programs but higher than out-patient drug free programs. A characteristic curve for attrition in traditional TCs shows that dropout is highest in the first 30 days, rises through 90 days and then decreases sharply.[15-16] Since traditional TC intervention lasts between 180 to 240 days, few admissions stay long enough to maximize treatment.

Research on correlates of retention has examined sociodemographic characteristics of clients; their attitudes, perceptions and beliefs; and/or circumstances related to their entry into treatment.[5,7,8,17-19] However, as Condelli and De Leon[10] report, no client profile has been found that strongly predicts retention in TCs or in any other drug treatment program.

For TCs, De Leon and Jainchill[20] hypothesize that four perceptual factors singularly or in combination significantly influence retention. These factors are circumstances (external reasons that influence an individual to seek treatment); motivation (an individual's internal reasons for change); readiness (an individual's perception that treatment is needed); and, suitability (an individual's perception that the treatment is appropriate for his/her needs). Motivation for treatment has long been considered important to entering and staying in treatment.[21-25] Pfeiffer, Feurlein and Brenk-Schulte[19] use the term "willingness" to characterize an array of variables thought to influence entry into and retention in treatment.

THE ASSET PROJECT

Arizona Settlement Services for Education and Transition (ASSET) was a three year project funded by the National Institute on Alcohol Abuse and Alcoholism to intervene with homeless adult drug users. Using a modified therapeutic community approach, ASSET's goals were to (1) decrease alcohol and/or drug use; (2) increase employability; and, (3) improve residential stability. The traditional TC model was modified to a 4 month program and included a residential and non-residential setting. The process of TC treatment remained intact but was accelerated to account for shorter duration of intervention.

The core of the intervention for both the residential and non-residential setting was a curriculum designed to examine, educate and affect substance use, housing and employment. The curriculum provided at least eight hours per week of contact between the homeless person and the intervention staff, allowing for didactic presentations, group work, individual counseling, retreats, community activities and social interaction. The curriculum was delivered by demonstrators trained in TC principles, who were often recovering addicts who completed treatment in a TC. The residential program provided services in a group home while services for the non-residential program were provided at a community center open 14-16 hours a day.

Three assumptions were made by ASSET staff as the intervention was developed and implemented. The first assumption was that the living conditions of a homeless drug user, including drug use, alcohol use, unstable housing and/or lack of income would influence his/her perceived willingness for treatment. The second assumption was that perceived willingness for treatment would relate to length of time in treatment. The last assumption was that living conditions on entry in ASSET, perceived willingness on entry and time in treatment would influence living conditions after leaving ASSET. This paper reports on analyses testing those assumptions.

METHODS

Sample: Eligibility criteria for ASSET were (1) at least 18 years of age; (2) homeless as defined by the McKinney Act; (3) reported an alcohol and/or drug problem; (4) did not use psychotropic medications; and, (5) agreed to random assignment to the residential or non-residential program. A nonequivalent comparison group, who met eligibility criteria one through four but refused treatment with ASSET, was also recruited.

Homeless adult drug users were recruited through street outreach, presentations to clients at homeless shelters, referrals from social service agencies, referrals from the criminal justice system, and by self-referral. Screening for eligibility occurred at the point of initial contact and was done by either intervention or research staff. Homeless persons not meeting eligibility criteria were told of other treatment services available in the community. Homeless persons, who met criteria, were informed of ASSET's research and intervention protocols. If an individual chose not to participate in the intervention, she/he was told about the comparison group and encouraged to take part in the research. This project was approved by the Institutional Review Board, University of Arizona.

Three hundred and fifty-eight homeless adults participated in the intervention and 136 in the comparison group. Sociodemographic characteristics for the intervention and comparison groups were similar. For the total sample, 89% were male; approximately 65% were less than 40 years of age; and, 40% were minorities including Blacks, Native Americans and Mexican Americans. Alcohol was the most problematic substance for over half of the sample followed by crack/cocaine use (30%). Most (60%) drank alcohol more than 10 days out of the last 30 days. Approximately 35% had never received alcohol treatment and over 50% never received drug treatment. Approximately 66% had not worked in the last month. On the average, the sample had stable housing for only 10 out of the previous 60 days. Half of the sample had been homeless twice in their lifetime and once in last five years.

Procedures: Once the choice to participate in the intervention or the comparison group was made, baseline interviews were conducted. Eligible persons agreeing to treatment were told that responses to the questionnaires would not influence their acceptance into the program nor their random assignment to the residential or non-residential setting. All questionnaires were administered by trained interviewers. No data were shared with the intervention staff.

Follow-up interviews were conducted at two, four, seven, ten and thirteen months after baseline. Intervention and comparison group members were paid $10.00 for time spent in the baseline interview and up to $25.00 for the follow-ups.

Measures: For data reported here, De Leon and Jainchill's[20] Motivation, Readiness and Suitability Scale (MRS) measured perceived willingness for treatment at baseline. Living conditions at baseline and at follow-up were measured using single items and a composite score from the Addiction Severity Index[26] and a composite score from the Personal History Form.[27] Length of time in treatment (retention) was measured as the number of days in ASSET from enrollment to discharge or drop out. Participants received no ASSET services after discharge (defined as completion of program) or drop out (defined as missing five or more continuous days of the program).

The MRS is a 42 item, five point Likert scale anchored with responses "strongly agree" and "strongly disagree". In ASSET, each item was read by an interviewer and the participant answered using one of the five possible responses or indicated "not applicable." The motivation subscale (17 items) measures internal reasons for change that can be positive (e.g., "I know I have to make changes in myself to get my life together") or negative ("I am afraid I will end up dead if I don't stop drinking or using drugs"). The readiness subscale (nine items) measures perceived need for formal treatment as opposed to self-directed change or assistance from significant others. A typical item in the readiness subscale is "Basically, I don't see any other choice for help at this time except some kind of treatment." The suitability subscale (16 items) measures an individual's perception of the appropriateness of the TC treatment model for him/herself. Example items for suitability are "I am willing to sever street ties for awhile if it will help me in treatment" and "I really do need to be completely alcohol/drug free in order to live successfully." The MRS is summated for a total scale score and for three subscale scores.

De Leon and Jainchill's Circumstances Subscale (CS), which measures losses (such as in relationships, family, support, job, school status or money) and fears (such as jail, injury, violence, suicide and death) was not used. Many homeless adults have already experienced those losses and lived with those fears. The CS, as constructed by De Leon and Jainchill, would not likely be sensitive to the losses and fears that drive homeless adult drug users to treatment.

In the initial test of the CMRS, De Leon and Jainchill[20] reported that seven items on the motivation subscale, seven items on readiness and eight items on suitability correlated significantly with 30 day retention in a residential TC. Smith and Simpson[28] found adequate reliability for the CMRS and three factors which were consistent with the conceptually defined domains.

Using the Addiction Severity Index (ASI), frequency of drug use was measured by summing responses to questions on consumption of ten street drugs including marijuana, cocaine, crack, heroin, opiates, hallucinogens, inhalants, barbiturates, sedative, and amphetamines. Each question asked "In the last 30 days, how many days did you use (name of drug)?" Possible responses for this measure were from zero to 300, ranging from no use of street drugs to use of all drugs on all 30 days. Using the same 30 day drug consumption question, days of any alcohol use were recorded. Responses from the ASI to "In the last 30 days, how many days were you paid for working?" measured employment.

To measure housing status, a composite from the Personal History Form (PHF) was created. The PHF asks "How many nights in the past 60 nights did you stay at (some location)?" Nights spent at locations that implied a housed condition (such as in own SRO, own domicile, parent/

guardian's domicile, treatment program, recovery program, or correctional facility) were summed.

Drug and alcohol use as well as employment and housing status were measured at baseline. Outcome measures for the four variables were computed by subtracting the baseline score from a follow-up score. Thus, an outcome was change in the frequency of a behavior. Desired outcomes of ASSET would be less drug and alcohol use as well as more days housed and employed at follow-up.

Not all treatment and comparison group members completed the follow-ups as scheduled. To obtain a follow-up measure on as many people as possible, scores on the seven month follow-up interview were used if available. If the seven month follow-up interview was not done, scores obtained from the ten month were used or if the ten month was not available, the 13 month interview was used. Under these conditions, 239 (54%) persons had follow-up measures and 202 (46%) had no follow-ups.

Statistical Analyses: The two statistical software packages used in these analyses were EQS[29] and SAS.[30] The data were subjected to a multivariate causal analysis using factor analytic structural equations modeling. A factor analytic structural equations model consists of two major components, a "measurement" model and a "structural" model. The measurement model is essentially confirmatory factor analysis, wherein a number of directly observed variables (indicators) are related to a smaller set of hypothetical constructs (latent variables or common factors) presumed to be underlying the correlations between them. For the purposes of this study, this procedure is superior to traditional exploratory factor analysis in that the exploratory procedure derives the multivariate constructs empirically from the correlations between indicators. Thus, exploratory factor analysis runs the risk of capitalizing upon chance associations and of equivocal *post hoc* interpretation of the factors.[31] Exploratory factor analysis is better suited for the generation rather than the testing of hypotheses. Instead, confirmatory factor analysis (CFA) permits the theoretical specification of the latent constructs as *a priori* hypotheses to be tested against correlational data. By the exclusive prior assignment of each indicator to theoretically specified constructs, CFA also reduces the number of factor loadings needed and thus, enhances the efficiency of parameter estimation. Because of multicollinearity, common factors were constructed for the three hypothetical latent variables of motivation, readiness and suitability.

Specifically, CFA tested the hypothesis that motivation, readiness and suitability were indeed well formed by the items in the scale. Since motivation, readiness and suitability were hypothetically correlated, the three factors were then considered for a higher order factor. The higher order construct was labelled willingness for treatment.

The structural component of the model is essentially a path analysis between the latent constructs that were produced by the factor analysis. Path analysis or structural equations modeling consists of imposing a restricted set of causal pathways, also specified *a priori*, and testing them against the correlations between constructs. Structural equations modeling permits the modeling of factor intercorrelations by any combination of direct, indirect, spurious and residual effects.[32]

In this study, the hypothesized direct effects were from the baseline score on a variable to willingness, from willingness to retention, from willingness to the change score at follow-up, from retention to the change score, and from the baseline to the change score. One hypothesized indirect path was from willingness through retention to each change score. This path analysis consisted of a multisample Generalized Least Squares causal model. Multisample analysis was required because follow-up data were missing on many subjects. Instead of deleting those cases with missing data, a simultaneous analysis kept those missing cases in and made the factor loadings as well as path coefficients equal for both follow-up and no follow-up groups. The Lagrange multiplier test was used to confirm that the constraints were equal to each other for the two groups.

To confirm that the group with follow-up data and the group without were similar for all baseline measures, a series of ANOVAs was run. ANOVA tested differences in means on baseline scores, motivation, readiness, suitability, and willingness for the two groups. For these univariate analyses, the factor scores were estimated by unit weighting.[31] PROC STANDARD in SAS was used to standardize the items. Next, the standardized items were averaged to get an estimate of the three lower order factors of motivation, readiness and suitability. The three lower order factors were then standardized and averaged to yield the higher order factor of willingness.

RESULTS

The Final Model: Figure 1 displays the factor analytic structural equations model. In this figure, the statistically significant causal pathways ($p \leq 0.05$) are represented as solid arrows while the nonsignificant causal pathways are represented by broken arrows. Both factor loadings and causal pathways are expressed as standardized regression coefficients (beta weights). The chi-square value for this model was 3014.608 (df = 2294) and was statistically significant ($p < 0.001$), indicating that the model did

FIGURE 1. Factor analytic structural equations model for baseline scores on four behaviors, motivation, readiness, suitability, willingness, retention, and change scores at follow-up, including significant and nonsignificant pathways.

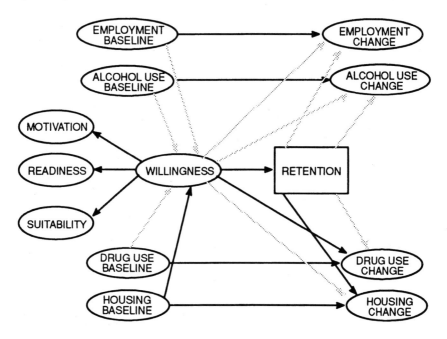

not perfectly predict all the covariances between the variables. However, all three of the practical fit indices for the model were highly acceptable. The normed Bentler-Bonett Fit Index was 0.983, the nonnormed Bentler-Bonett Fit Index was 0.996 and the Comparative Fit Index was 0.996. Such indices of fit exceeding 0.90 are considered acceptable for practical purposes.[33] The substantive aspects of this model are now discussed.

The Measurement Model: Lower order common factors were constructed for the motivation, readiness and suitability subscales of the MRS. Table 1 presents a summary of the findings. In this table, the content of an item is reflected in two or more key words. For motivation, loadings for the 17 items ranged from −0.006 to 0.882 with one item having a negative and 16 items having positive correlations with the factor. For readiness, factor loadings of the nine items ranged from 0.610 to 0.948. For suitability, loadings of the 16 items ranged from 0.280 to 0.867. All positive factor loadings or correlations were statistically significant.

TABLE 1. Item Loadings on Motivation, Readiness and Suitability.

Item Content	Motivation	Readiness	Suitability
Serious Problem	0.882		
Cause Of Problems	0.735		
Stay Off Drugs	0.805		
Don't Like Self	0.796		
Can't Control Life	0.818		
Life Worse	0.813		
End Up Dead	0.737		
Make Changes	0.682		
Important To Stop	0.850		
Make Changes	− 0.006		
Other Problems	0.371		
Family Pressure	0.566		
Family Influence	0.759		
Continue Use	0.820		
Drugs No Problem	0.620		
Lost Everything	0.652		
Hurt People	0.647		
Stop Anytime		0.699	
Ready For Treatment		0.822	
Do Anything		0.706	
No Other Choice		0.902	
Need Treatment		0.856	
Try Other Treatment		0.610	
Can't Do Myself		0.861	
Enter Soon		0.948	
Another Chance		0.621	

TABLE 1 (continued)

	Motivation	Readiness	Suitability
Sever Family Ties			0.683
Sever Street Ties			0.867
Right Approach			0.805
New Environment			0.700
Change Attitude			0.688
Drug Free			0.884
Other Treatment			0.280
Sacrifices To Stay			0.496
No Serious Problems			0.698
Change A Lot			0.381
Stay Away From Users			0.754
Tried Other Treatment			0.301
Need This Program			0.832
Fears About Program			0.386
Demands Of Program			0.452
Stay Long			0.718

CFA confirmed the hypothesized factor structure of the MRS. Pearson correlation coefficients between the motivation, readiness and suitability subscales were all greater than 0.79 and significant at a p value less than 0.000. Similarly, correlations between each subscale and the total MRS scale were high ranging from 0.85 to 0.94. The factors labelled motivation, readiness and suitability that were identified in CFA were also correlated. The motivation factor correlated to the readiness factor at 0.58 and to the suitability factor at 0.55. The readiness factor correlated at 0.90 with the suitability factor. This pattern of relationships suggested that the three subscales were tapping into another common factor.

CFA confirmed the higher order factor (see Figure 1). Loading of the motivation factor on the higher order construct was 0.947. Loading of the readiness factor was 0.981 and suitability factor was 0.981 on the higher order construct. The higher order construct was labelled willingness to encompass motivation, readiness, and suitability.

The very high, nearly perfect, correlations between the three lower order factors and the higher order construct provide strong evidence against the discriminate validity of the three separate subscales. Parsimony also advocates for the use of only the higher order construct in analyses. The structural model discussed below used willingness as a predictor of retention and project outcomes.

The Structural Model: The structural model linking baseline measures on four behaviors, willingness, retention and changes in the four behaviors at follow-up is shown in Figure 1. For the full structural model, eight out of the 17 hypothesized direct causal pathways were statistically significant. Two hypothesized indirect paths to the change scores were also significant. The structural model is now discussed looking at pathways from left to right.

Only one significant relation was found between a behavior at baseline and willingness. For the homeless drug user, more stable housing at baseline increased his/her willingness for treatment. Days of employment, alcohol use or drug use at baseline had no relation to willingness.

For each of the four behaviors, there was a significant, negative causal pathway from baseline to the change score at follow-up. This finding suggested that the higher the frequency of a behavior at baseline, the smaller the change at follow-up. Thus, the more employment days reported at baseline, the less change in employment at follow-up from that baseline score. Similar statements can be made for the relationship of baseline alcohol use, drug use or days housed to its change score.

A significant, positive path from willingness to retention implied that the more willing the homeless drug users were for treatment at baseline, the longer he/she stayed in ASSET. Willingness also had one significant direct path to change in behavior. More willingness for treatment at baseline related to more change in drug use at follow-up.

Although mediated by retention, willingness had an effect on housing change. This indirect pathway suggested that the more willing a homeless drug user was at baseline, the greater the housing change at follow-up. Willingness had no other significant direct or indirect effects on the four change scores.

Longer retention related directly to more change in days of stable housing. Contrary to our expectations, retention or length of time in treatment had no direct effect on change in employment, alcohol use or drug use at follow-up.

This multivariate causal model explained 23% of the variance for change in employment, 61% for change in alcohol days, 67% for change in drug days and 37% for change in housing. The Lagrange multiplier tests were all nonsignificant confirming equality constraints. The ANOVAs found no significant differences between groups with and without follow-up data for the baseline measures.

DISCUSSION

The purpose of this study was to test assumptions made in the development and implementation of the ASSET project. Program staff hypothesized that pre-existing living conditions of homeless adult drug users would influence their perceived willingness for TC treatment as well as outcomes of treatment. Willingness, specifically motivation, readiness and perceived suitability for treatment, would influence length of time in ASSET and treatment outcomes. Lastly, length of time in treatment would influence outcomes. Data were subjected to a multivariate causal analysis using factor analytic structural equations modeling. From this analysis, several hypotheses were supported.

The measurement model confirmed the hypothesized factor structure of De Leon and Jainchill's Motivation, Readiness and Suitability Scale (MRS) but found no discriminate validity among the three subscales. A higher order factor, labelled willingness, fit the observed data well. From the structural model, willingness had a significant, positive relationship to retention. This finding is consistent with the literature on motivation and time in treatment.[21-25] The strength of the relationship found in this study is slightly larger than correlates reported previously for long term residential treatment.[20-21]

Willingness had strong evidence for its construct and predictive validity. The composite MRS scale may be useful in screening applicants for TC treatment and perhaps, in monitoring intent to stay in treatment for program participants. From other analyses of the ASSET program, the non-equivalent comparison group had lower scores on the MRS than those entering treatment; and, ASSET participants who stayed in treatment longer than 30 days had higher MRS scores than those dropping out before one month.[34] In ASSET, willingness was measured only at baseline. However, qualitative research findings from our study suggest that willingness changes during treatment and may intensify, diminish or remain stable over time.[34] Those homeless adult drug users maintaining low levels of willingness or reporting less willingness as treatment time increased were more likely to drop out. Large scale, prospective studies of willingness on entry and during TC treatment are needed.

The structural model supported several hypothesized relationships. Only one baseline living condition, nights of stable housing positively influenced willingness for TC treatment. More hypothesized causal pathways were significant for change in housing than for the other three outcomes. Baseline score for housing as well as retention directly influenced housing change. Likewise, a path from the baseline score to willingness continuing through retention significantly influenced housing change. These findings are reasonable given that homelessness was the primary criterion for entry into ASSET. Housing, a basic human need, was the overwhelming reason our sample sought TC treatment. For those homeless drug users who experienced stable housing in the previous sixty days, the drive to continue a housed condition was high. Drug use, alcohol use and unemployment may have been secondary considerations in seeking treatment. Another explanation could be that the actual problems associated with the other three behaviors at baseline were less than those related to homelessness. Merely the presence, not the degree of a perceived drug and/or alcohol problem, met eligibility criterion. Unemployment was not a necessary criterion for entry into ASSET. The homelessness of these adult drug users limits generalizability of these findings. Drug users, who have met their basic need for stable housing, might view alcohol use, drug use and/or employment issues as strong primary reasons for seeking TC treatment.

Structural modeling found significant, negative relationships between baseline and change on employment, alcohol use, drug use and housing. Two explanations should be considered. First, it is not unreasonable to argue that homeless adults with more problems at baseline (less days employed, more alcohol use, more drug use, less housed) would be less likely to substantially change their living conditions during the time to follow. Also, it is not unreasonable to hypothesize that homeless adults with fewer problems would be more likely to change over time. The second explanation is regression towards the mean which may be evidenced by inflated negative autoregression effects between baseline and change scores. Since our findings demonstrated negative effects, regression towards the mean cannot be ruled out entirely. Nevertheless, its existence as a partial explanation of the structural relations between our baseline and change scores would not compromise our major conclusions. This study was explicitly modeled as a non-equivalent groups design.[35] All treatment effects were statistically controlled for the effects of baseline scores, whether extreme or otherwise. Furthermore, the effects of other baseline measures on willingness were also assessed. Thus, if regression towards the mean did occur, it could have no biasing effect upon our principal findings.

In the structural model, retention had no significant path to employment, alcohol or drug change at follow-up. This finding may imply that treatment had no influence on these outcomes but that interpretation is incorrect. Rather, retention in treatment had no effect on outcomes. This finding has two possible explanations. First, the curriculum used in the ASSET intervention was delivered over a four month period of time. Homeless drug users entering ASSET began the curriculum not at its start but at a point in its cycle. Each drug user probably had a slightly different start on the curriculum and depending on length of time in the program, different experiences in treatment. Thus, retention and treatment content interact in influencing outcomes. The relationships among retention, treatment characteristics and outcomes need examination. The second explanation for retention failing to correlate with three outcomes regards the TC process used in this program. ASSET modified the traditional TC by shortening the time in treatment, accelerating the process and working in a non-traditional setting. Possibly one or more of these modifications changed the TC treatment process enough so that significant effects on alcohol and drug use could not be achieved in four or fewer months. This explanation is being explored in the ASSET data.

REFERENCES

1. Allison M, Hubbard R. Drug abuse treatment process: A review of the literature. Int J Addict. 1985; 20:1321-1345.

2. Joe G, Simpson D. Retention in treatment of drug users admitted to treatment during 1971-1972. In Sells S, Simpson D, eds. Studies in the effectiveness of treatment of drug abuse. Cambridge, MA: Ballinger, 1974:253-324.

3. Hubbard R, Marsden M, Rachel J, Harwood H, Cavanaugh E, Ginzburg H. Drug abuse treatment: a national study of effectiveness. Chapel Hill: University of North Carolina Press, 1989.

4. Simpson S, Sells S. Effectiveness of treatment for drug abuse: an overview of the DARP research program. Adv Alcohol Subst Abuse. 1982; 2:7-29.

5. Siddall J, Conway G. Interactional variables associated with retention and success in residential drug treatment. Int J Addict. 1988; 23:1241-1254.

6. Simpson D. The relation of time spent in drug abuse treatment to post treatment outcomes. Am J Psychiatry. 1979; 136:1449-1453.

7. Craig R. Personality dimensions related to premature termination from an inpatient drug abuse treatment program. J Clin Psychol. 1984; 40:351-355.

8. Baekeland F, Lundwall L. Dropping out of treatment: a critical review. Psychol Bull. 1975; 82:738-783.

9. De Leon G, Schwartz S. The therapeutic community: what are the retention rates? Am J Drug Alcohol Abuse. 1984; 10:267-284.

10. Condelli W, De Leon G. Fixed and dynamic predictors of client retention in therapeutic communities. J Subst Abuse Treat. 1993; 10:11-16.

11. Condelli W, Dunteman G. Issues to consider when predicting retention in therapeutic communities. J Psychoactive Drugs. 1993; 25:239-244.

12. De Leon G, Wexler H, Jainchill N. The therapeutic community: success and improvement rates 5 years after treatment. Int J Addict. 1982; 17:703-747.

13. Simpson D. Treatment for drug abuse. Arch Gen Psychiatry. 1981; 38:875-880.

14. Bale R, VanStone W, Kuldau J, Enselsing T, Elashoff R, Zarcone V. Therapeutic communities vs. methadone maintenance: a prospective study of narcotic addiction treatment. Arch Gen Psychiatry. 1980; 37:179-183.

15. De Leon G. Retention in drug free therapeutic communities. In Pickens R, Leukefeld C, eds. Improving drug abuse treatment (NIDA Monograph 106). Washington, DC: US Government Printing Office, 1991:218-244.

16. De Leon G. The therapeutic community: status and evolution. Int J Addict. 1985; 20:823-844.

17. De Leon G. The therapeutic community: study of effectiveness (NIDA Monograph, No. ADM 84-1286). Washington, DC: US Government Printing Office, 1984.

18. De Leon G. Legal pressure in therapeutic communities. In Leukefeld C, Tims F, eds. Compulsory treatment of drug abuse: research and clinical practice (NIDA Monograph 86). Washington, DC: US Government Printing Office, 1988:160-177.

19. Pfeiffer W, Feuerlein W, Brenk-Schulte E. The motivation of alcohol dependents to undergo treatment. Drug Alcohol Depend. 1991; 29:87-95.

20. De Leon G, Jainchill N. Circumstances, motivation, readiness and suitability (CMRS) and correlates of treatment tenure. J Psychoactive Drugs. 1986; 8:203-208.

21. Simpson D, Joe G. Motivation as a predictor of early dropout. Psychother. 1993; 30:357-367.

22. Beckman J. An attributional analysis of alcoholics anonymous. J Stud Alcohol. 1980; 41:714-726.

23. Karoly P. Person variables in therapeutic change and development. In Karoly P, Steffer J, eds. Improving the long-term effects of psychotherapy. New York: Gardner, 1980: 195-261.

24. Cox W, Klinger E. Motivational model of alcohol use. J Abnorm Psychol. 1988; 97:168-180.

25. Miller W. Motivation for treatment: a review with special emphasis on alcoholism. Psychol Bull. 1985; 98:84-107.

26. McLellan A, Luborsky L, O'Brien C, Woody G. An improved diagnostic evaluation instrument for substance abuse patients: The addiction severity index. J of Nervous and Mental Disease. 1980; 168:26-33.

27. Barrow S, Hellman F, Lovell A, Plapinger D, Streuning E. Personal history form. Community Support Systems Evaluation Program. Epidemiology of Mental Disorders Research Department. New York: New York State Psychiatric Institute, 1985.

28. Smith S, Simpson D. Client assessment at drug abuse treatment intake for predicting tenure. Paper presented at the Southwestern Psychological Association Conference 1988.

29. Bentler P. EQS structural equations program manual. Los Angeles: BMDP Statistical Software, Inc., 1989.

30. SAS Institute, Inc. SAS language and procedures: Usage, Version 6, First Edition. Cary, NC: SAS Institute, 1989.

31. Gorsuch R. Factor analysis. Hillsdale, NJ: Lawrence Erlbaum, 1983.

32. James L, Mulaik S, Brett J. Causal analysis: Assumptions, models, and data. Beverly Hills, CA: Sage Publications, 1982.

33. Bentler P, Bonett, D. Significance tests and goodness of fit in the analysis of convariance structures. Psychol Bull. 1980; 88:588-606.

34. Erickson JR, Stevens S. The ASSET project: Process and outcomes of modified therapeutic community interventions among homeless adult drug users. (Final Report of Project Activities, NIAAA Grant U01 AA08788, 1994).

35. Cook T, Campbell D. Quasi-experimentation. Boston: Houghton Mifflin Company, 1979.

Evaluating Alternative Treatments for Homeless Substance-Abusing Men: Outcomes and Predictors of Success

Gerald J. Stahler, PhD
Thomas F. Shipley, Jr., PhD
David Bartelt, PhD
Joseph P. DuCette, PhD
Irving W. Shandler, MA, MSW

SUMMARY. The present study was designed to explore the relative efficacy of three types of service delivery intervention models for home-

Gerald J. Stahler is affiliated with the Department of Geography and Urban Studies, Thomas F. Shipley, Jr., is affiliated with the Department of Psychology, David Bartelt is affiliated with the Department of Geography and Urban Studies, Joseph P. DuCette is affiliated with the Department of Psychological Studies in Education, Temple University.

Irving W. Shandler is affiliated with Diagnostic and Rebilitation Center of Philadelphia.

Address correspondence to Gerald Stahler, PhD, Department of Geography and Urban Studies, 329 Gladfelter Hall (025-26), Temple University, Philadelphia, PA 19122.

The authors wish to thank Ellen Goss, Tom O'Malley, and the rest of the DRC staff, as well as the DRC clients who graciously participated in this study. The authors also acknowledge the excellent contributions made by Danielle Westcott, Alan Sockloff, and the Temple research assistants for all of their efforts in the conduct of the study.

Support for this project was provided in part by The National Institute on Alcohol Abuse and Alcoholism (NIAAA); Cooperative Agreement #AA 08802-02.

[Haworth co-indexing entry note]: "Evaluating Alternative Treatments for Homeless Substance-Abusing Men: Outcomes and Predictors of Success." Stahler, Gerald J., et al. Co-published simultaneously in the *Journal of Addictive Diseases* (The Haworth Medical Press, an imprint of The Haworth Press, Inc.) Vol. 14, No. 4, 1995, pp. 151-167; and: *The Effectiveness of Social Interventions for Homeless Substance Abusers* (ed: Gerald J. Stahler) The Haworth Medical Press, an imprint of The Haworth Press, Inc., 1995, pp. 151-167. Single or multiple copies of this article are available from The Haworth Document Delivery Service [1-800-342-9678; 9:00 a.m. - 5:00 p.m. (EST)].

151

less men with alcohol and/or drug problems: integrated comprehensive residential services provided at one site (Group 1); on-site shelter-based intensive case management with referrals to a community network of services (Group 2); and usual care shelter services with case management (Group 3). In addition to assessing the relative efficacy of these approaches in terms of drug and alcohol use, residential stability, economic and employment status, the project also sought to examine what personal factors best predicted successful outcomes for clients. Clients were assessed at baseline and approximately six months following discharge. All three treatment groups improved significantly over time in terms of reduced alcohol and cocaine use, increased employment, and increased stable housing, but no differential improvement was found among groups. Successful outcomes were predicted by lower recent and lifetime substance use, fewer prior treatment episodes, more stable housing at baseline, fewer incarcerations, and less social isolation. *[Article copies available from The Haworth Document Delivery Service: 1-800-342-9678.]*

While there has been considerable research conducted on treatment effectiveness for alcohol and drug abuse, relatively little is currently known about the effectiveness of interventions for *homeless* persons with alcohol and/or other drug abuse problems. Initial interventions with the homeless typically consist of providing shelter with minimal assistance to meet such other needs as medical treatment, detoxification, counseling, case management, or other services. As a result, some have advocated the need for providing more intensive service interventions, particularly case management that provides for continuous service planning, advocacy, benefits acquisition, and service linkages and monitoring.[1] Another approach is to offer comprehensive services at one site so that clients do not have to travel to a variety of settings for different services, and where continuity of care and integration of services is emphasized.

In September, 1990, Temple University in conjunction with the Diagnostic and Rehabilitation Center (DRC) of Philadelphia was awarded a demonstration grant from the National Institute of Alcohol Abuse and Alcoholism (NIAAA) to develop and assess the relative effectiveness of these alternative service approaches in the treatment of approximately 700 homeless, male polydrug users recruited from a large men's homeless shelter. Specifically, the present study was designed to explore the relative efficacy of three types of service delivery intervention models for homeless men with alcohol and/or drug problems: integrated comprehensive residential services provided at one site (Group 1); on-site shelter-based intensive case management, information, and referral services to a community network of programs (Group 2); and usual care shelter services with case management and referral (Group 3). In addition to assessing the relative efficacy of these approaches in terms of drug and alcohol use, residential stability, economic and employment status, the project also sought to examine what personal factors (demographic, social/psychological) best predict successful outcomes for these clients.

METHODS

The present study recruited clients over a period of 18 months from the Ridge Avenue Shelter, the largest men's homeless shelter in Philadelphia at the time of the study. All clients who entered the shelter during this period were screened for the following eligibility criteria for participation in the study: age 18 or older, stable mental health (no active psychosis or uncontrollable aggression), no profound mental retardation, and presence of a problem with alcohol and/or drug use. Of a total of 1731 potential subjects screened, 722, or 42%, were found eligible and willing to participate, and received baseline interviews. These clients were then randomly assigned to one of three treatment conditions: *Group 1*, a 6-month comprehensive, residential treatment program; *Group 2*, a 4- to 9-month shelter-based intensive case management program staffed primarily by peer counselors; and *Group 3*, a program of regular shelter services provided by city-staffed case managers who typically had very large case loads. Clients assigned to Group 1 remained in the shelter for several days, and then were transferred to the residential treatment facility. This program involved a variety of services, including individual counseling, group therapy, lectures, life skills preparation, job search skills training, and vocational and educational training. Particular emphasis was placed on participating in 12-step programs (Alcoholics Anonymous and Narcotics Anonymous).

Those assigned to Groups 2 and 3 remained in the shelter. The Group 2 program was an intensive case management program utilizing indigenous case managers who were often themselves involved in the recovery process. The case managers assisted clients in establishing linkages with community-based services to further promote sober and independent living. Caseloads tended to be approximately 15 clients per case manager. In addition, social workers provided aftercare services once the clients left the shelter.

Those clients assigned to Group 3 received the usual city services provided at the shelter by degreed social worker case managers. Typically, clients received traditional case management services in the shelter, with caseloads of roughly 50-75 per case manager. The primary responsibility of the case managers was to broker ancillary or supportive services for clients, and assist them in acquiring stable housing. Case managers developed an initial service plan for each client and then referred him to appropriate services. Unlike Groups 1 and 2, there was no specific programmatic graduation or end point for clients. Group 3 was considered the comparison group for the purpose of assessing the effectiveness of the two experimental treatment groups (Groups 1 and 2).

Clients were assessed at three points in time: at intake or baseline, at discharge, and approximately 6 months following discharge. Since the six month post-discharge data are considered the true test of program effectiveness, only these data will be reported in this paper. The major assessment measures included the Addiction Severity Index (ASI),[2] a revised version of the Personal History Form[3] to assess residential history, and the Client Satisfaction Questionnaire.[4] A more complete programmatic description can be found in Shipley et al.[5] and Stahler et al.[6]

Of the 722 clients who entered the study and received baseline assessments, 76% were located and interviewed approximately 6 months after discharge. Clients who received follow-up interviews were compared with clients who did not on a number of baseline variables to examine the selection bias of the follow-up sample. No differences between groups (p < .05) were found on any of the variables assessed, including alcohol and cocaine use (recent and lifetime), housing history, and age. While we cannot be assured of the equivalence of groups at follow-up because of the possible differential exposure to treatment as well as to other post-baseline experiences which might influence outcomes, we can assume that the clients who received follow-up interviews are representative of the entire sample of clients at baseline.

Whereas *study* attrition was quite low given the mobility of this population, *treatment* attrition was quite high as has been typically found by many programs which serve substance abusers. Of those assigned to Group 1, only 14% completed the program, compared to 29% of those assigned to Group 2. However, more than half of the clients who dropped out of treatment in Group 1 did so *prior* to beginning the program. Considering only those clients in Group 1 who actually began treatment, 26% graduated–a figure comparable to that of Group 2. Because Group 3, the comparison group, was not a formally constructed program, there was no comparable services end point to classify as program completion or graduation.

RESULTS

Description of the Sample at Baseline

Table 1 presents some of the major characteristics of the sample at baseline. Overall, the data depict a sample of young African-American (91%)

TABLE 1. Baseline Characteristics of Sample.

	Group 1: Residential Treatment (n = 220)	Group 2: Intensive Case Mgt (n = 200)	Group 3: Usual Shelter Svs. (n = 302)	Total (n = 722)
Mean Age	32.1	32.8	32.8	32.6
Race				
% White	8	6	5	6
% Black	91	92	92	92
% Other	1	3	3	2
Education				
% < high school	47	42	48	46
% high school	42	40	39	40
% some college	11	19	13	14
Marital Status				
% currently married	7	5	7	7
% previously married	25	33	29	29
% never married	68	62	64	65
% Veteran	18	28	24	23
Usual Employment Past Year				
% full time	32	39	39	37
% part time	30	24	25	26
% unemployed	37	38	36	37
Primary problem substance				
% cocaine	76	76	77	77
% alcohol	21	22	18	20
% other	3	2	5	3
Days cocaine use past 30 days	11	11	11	11
Days intoxicated with alcohol, past 30 days	10	6	9	8
Number times homeless				
% one episode	55	50	46	50
% two episodes	24	26	28	26
% three or more	21	24	26	24
Mean % of nights homeless of past 60 (includes living on street, shelter, or doubled up)	51	53	52	52

men, who for the most part use crack cocaine as well as alcohol. Most have never been married and nearly half never completed high school. For half the sample, the present episode was their first experience of homelessness, and over three fourths of the sample have had less than three episodes of homelessness. To ascertain the equivalence of groups at baseline, the three treatment groups were compared on a variety of variables concerning demographic characteristics, drug use, housing status, employment, and other psychosocial domains using multiple analyses of variance (MANOVA) and Chi squares where appropriate. In general, the three groups were found to be equivalent on all variables except for alcohol use during the 30 days prior to baseline assessment on which Group 2 clients reported less use than the other two groups (p < .05).

Outcome Results

Statistical analyses were guided by the goals of the research project and focused on two areas: (1) assessing differential outcomes by treatment group; (2) predicting outcomes across groups as a result of individual background factors.

We had initially hypothesized that there would be group differences on outcomes showing that residential treatment was more effective than shelter-based intensive case management services, which in turn would be more effective than clients receiving usual shelter services. Overall, the present study found very little differential effectiveness among these treatment groups. Using repeated measures analyses of variance, we found no significant differences on outcomes (p < .05) among the treatment groups on substance use, housing stability, employment, or psychological status. However, the results from a three group discriminant function analysis on the 18 items of the Client Satisfaction Questionnaire indicated that clients were much more satisfied (p = .002) with the services provided in the treatment groups (Groups 1 and 2) compared to Group 3.

The only other differences among treatment groups involved analyses comparing subgroups based on entry and exit status within each of the major treatment groups. Comparisons were made across groups between those who never started treatment, those who started and then dropped out, and those who went straight through the program and graduated. Repeated measures ANOVAs revealed that those clients who went straight through treatment in Groups 1 and 2 (as opposed to dropping out or being discharged) improved more on alcohol use and housing stability than clients in Group 3 (p < .05). However, they were not different in terms of cocaine use, employment status, or psychological problems.

Perhaps by far the most striking findings were the dramatic positive outcomes found across *all* three groups over time even though there was no differential improvement among groups. As shown in Table 2, on average, 58% of the clients who used alcohol as their primary substance of abuse, and 74% of cocaine users reported that they were abstinent for the prior 30 days at follow-up, yielding a total abstinence rate for users of these substances of 71%. Across groups, all outcome variables showed significant improvement ($p < .05$) between baseline and follow-up, including such indicators as number of days of stable housing during the 60 days prior to the follow-up interview, recent alcohol and cocaine use, money

TABLE 2. Summary of the Major Outcome Variables.

VARIABLE	PRETEST	POSTTEST	% CHANGE
Stable Housing (days out of last 30)	20.53	24.79	+21%
Literal Homelessness (days out of last 30)	11.59	8.13	−30%
Alcohol Use (days out of last 30)	10.52	3.74	−64%
Money Spent for Alcohol ($ per month)	$39.30	$21.83	−44%
Cocaine Use (days out of last 30)	11.88	3.16	−73%
Money for Drugs ($ per month)	$405.82	$110.74	−73%
Money from Employment ($ per month)	$185.86	$317.80	+71%
Money from Illegal Sources ($ per month)	$244.16	$62.63	−74%
Days paid for working (days out of last 30)	5.06	8.76	+73%
Days of illegal activity (days out of last 30)	3.15	1.07	−66%
Serious conflicts with family (days out of last 30)	3.55	2.11	−41%
Psychological Troubles (days out of last 30)	12.56	6.13	−51%
Cocaine Abstinence prior 30 days (for primary cocaine users)	0%	74%	NA
Alcohol Abstinence prior 30 days (for primary alcohol users)	0%	58%	NA

from employment, days paid for working, serious conflicts with family members, and days experiencing psychological problems.

Predicting Successful Outcomes

A second set of analyses were performed to ascertain if individual differences at baseline could predict outcomes at follow-up using a series of hierarchical multiple regression analyses. Since there were virtually no differences between treatment groups on outcomes, all three groups were combined to examine successful outcomes regardless of treatment group. The criterion variables used in these analyses represented the primary outcome domains of cocaine and alcohol use during the 30 days prior to the follow-up interview, number of days employed and number of days living in stable housing during the preceding 30 days. Since the number of possible predictor variables was quite large, it was decided to analyze the variables in waves. That is, logically related variables were entered into the regression equation in a hierarchical fashion. Those variables which were significant in one wave were carried forward into the next wave and so on until all of the waves had been analyzed. As a final analysis, all of the variables that had been significant at any point were entered into a final regression equation from which the final multiple R was computed.

For all four of the regressions, the variable sets were identical as follows:

Wave 1: demographic variables (e.g., age, education, marital status);
Wave 2: lifetime variables related to the specific criterion variable being analyzed (e.g., for alcohol, lifetime alcohol use and lifetime alcohol treatment episodes);
Wave 3: past 30 day behavior related to the criterion (e.g., for alcohol, amount of alcohol consumed in the 30 days prior to program entry);
Wave 4: lifetime and past 30 day behavior related to the other three criterion variables (e.g., for alcohol, lifetime and 30 day cocaine use);
Wave 5: legal problems (e.g., number of times incarcerated in lifetime);
Wave 6: family and social issues (e.g., current living arrangements; problems with family members in 30 days prior to treatment);
Wave 7: psychological state at baseline (e.g., depression and mood state).

Table 3 summarizes these regressions by presenting the variables found to significantly predict the above outcomes across groups, the level of significance, and the sign of the beta weight derived from the initial regression analysis.

Overall, although all four of the regression analyses were significant at the .05 level, the amount of variance accounted for by these equations (adjusted R^2) was moderately low, ranging between 8% and 21%, and thus should be viewed with some caution. It is evident, however, that alcohol and cocaine abstinence are more predictable than either employment or housing with the adjusted R^2 for the two substance variables almost twice as great as for employment or housing.

Younger age and greater education were significantly related to reduced alcohol use, but not to any of the other criterion variables. Subjects who had been in a controlled environment (primarily a treatment environment) during the 30 days prior to program entry were using less cocaine. However, overall, the criterion variables were not strongly predicted by demographic variables.

The only criterion variable predicted by lifetime variables was cocaine use. Clients who had a longer history of cocaine use and a greater number of times in drug detoxification programs tended to be less successful in reducing cocaine use. That is, long term, chronic users were less likely to be abstinent from cocaine.

The results from the third wave suggest that recent functioning prior to baseline is predictive of posttreatment outcomes. That is, the better the subject had been doing prior to treatment in a specific domain, the better the subject was doing at the posttest on that same variable. For example, subjects who had been using less cocaine during the 30 days prior to baseline tended to use less cocaine at follow-up. Clients who had been employed for more days in the 30 days preceding entry into treatment tended to have more days employment at follow-up; and clients who had spent more time in stable housing prior to treatment were experiencing more stable housing following treatment.

In addition, baseline variables in one outcome domain seemed to predict criterion variables in other domains. For example, alcohol use was predicted by such baseline variables as lower recent cocaine use, lower recent polydrug use, fewer prior drug treatment episodes, and a greater perceived importance of obtaining drug treatment. Similarly, cocaine abstinence was predicted by less recent alcohol use, but greater lifetime use. This may be indicative of the fact that some clients who were "pure" alcoholics would most likely have longer lifetime use of alcohol than non-chronic alcoholics, and may therefore have a tendency to use cocaine to a lesser degree at follow-up. Greater recent polydrug use was predictive of poorer outcomes on alcohol use, employment, and stable housing at follow-up.

Criminal activity also seems to play a role in predicting outcomes, at least for alcohol and cocaine use. Recent illegal activity was associated with

TABLE 3. Significance Levels and Beta Signs for Baseline Variables Predicting Outcomes.

	Reduced Alcohol Use		Reduced Cocaine Use		Days Paid for Work		Days of Stable Housing	
	p of beta	beta sign	p of beta	beta sign	p of beta	beta sign	p of beta	beta sign
WAVE 1: Demographic Variables								
Age	.023	−						
Education	.041	+	.030	+				
Days in controlled environment								
WAVE 2: Lifetime Variables Specifically Related to Criterion Variable								
Lifetime cocaine use	NA		.002	−	NA		NA	
Number of times in drug detox program			.003	−	NA		NA	
WAVE 3: Past 30 days at Baseline Specifically Related to Criterion Variable								
Days treated for alc/drugs in past 30 days	.002	−	NA		NA		NA	
Cocaine use in past 30 days	NA		.031	−	NA		NA	
Days paid for work in past 30 days	NA		NA		.020	+	NA	
Stable housing in past 30 days							.003	+
WAVE 4: Lifetime and 30 day Behaviors Related to Any of the Other Criterion Variables								
Cocaine use in past 30 days	.031	−	NA		.031	−		
More than one substance per day in past 30	.052	−						

Predictor	β	p	β	p	β	p	β	p
Number of times treated for drug abuse	—	.022		NA			—	.023
Importance of drug treatment presently receiving	+	.016		NA				
Alcohol use in past 30 days		NA	—	.011				
Lifetime alcohol use		NA	+	.000				
Stable housing in past 30 days					+	.019		
WAVE 5: Legal Issues								
Days of illegal activity, past 30 days	—	.000	—	.004			—	.018
Money from illegal sources	—	.004						
Number of incarcerations/lifetime			—	.012				
WAVE 6: Family and Social								
How troubled by problems with others	+	.016	+	.021			—	.006
Free time spent alone					+	.034		
Serious family conflicts in past 30 days			—	.017				
WAVE 7: Psychological Variables								
Trouble with controlling violent behavior	—	.051						
Depression					—	.007		
How troubled by psychological problems							—	.003
Adjusted R²		.174		.211		.113		.085
p		.000		.000		.018		.042

Notes:

Numbers in table represent exact p levels.

Variables listed in each wave are only those found to be significant. Non-significant predictors are not listed.

+ = positive beta weight

− = negative beta weight

NA = predictor in this wave not relevant to the criterion variable.

increased alcohol use and cocaine use at posttest, and the number of lifetime incarcerations was negatively associated with stable housing.

Several variables involving interpersonal relations were significantly associated with outcomes. In general, the greater the degree of interpersonal conflicts reported at baseline, the better the outcomes. For example, those *more* troubled by problems with others used less cocaine and alcohol at follow-up. This might be because those men who are using substances to a higher degree are not troubled by problems with others because they are so involved with their addictive substances and may not be as involved in relating to others, positively or negatively. Indeed, there is some support for this explanation in that those with a tendency to spend most of their free time alone are likely to be using more cocaine at follow-up. Spending free time alone was also associated with less stable housing situations at follow-up. Another variable measuring family relationships which was significantly associated with an outcome variable was days of serious family conflicts at baseline. The greater the family conflicts, the greater the number of days of employment at follow-up. This may be because those who are relatively successful in obtaining employment are more involved with their families, even if they are conflicted relationships.

Finally, only a few psychological variables were significantly associated with the criterion variables. Recent depression was inversely related to the number of days employed at the follow-up, and how troubled by psychological problems was inversely related to stable housing. Subjects who had less trouble controlling violent behavior at baseline were experiencing greater success regarding alcohol use. Overall, however, the subjects' psychological state at baseline appeared to be only modestly associated with outcomes at the posttest.

To ascertain if there was a differential effect of the three treatment interventions on client subgroups, separate hierarchical multiple regressions were computed for the two treatment groups and the comparison group in an identical format as the regressions presented above. In general, the pattern of beta weights from these regressions were similar to the pattern from the total group analyses. Therefore, these data suggest that various subgroups of clients did not respond differentially to the three treatments.

In summary, less alcohol use at follow-up was moderately predicted by younger age and greater educational attainment, less prior drug and alcohol treatment, lower recent cocaine and polydrug use, greater perceived importance for obtaining drug treatment, less illegal activity, a greater feeling of being troubled by problems with others, and less trouble controlling violent behavior. Less cocaine use at follow-up was associated with more days spent in a controlled environment during the past 30, fewer years of cocaine use, fewer number of times in drug detoxification programs, lower recent cocaine use, lower recent alcohol use but greater lifetime alcohol use, less criminal activity and incarcerations, less tendency to spend one's free time alone, and feeling more troubled by problems with others.

Employment and stable housing at follow-up were both predicted by fewer variables which explained a relatively low amount of the variance for each criterion. Employment was predicted modestly by recent employment and stable housing prior to baseline, recent serious family conflicts, and a lower degree of recent polydrug use and depression. Stable housing was very modestly predicted by recent stable housing at baseline, less recent polydrug use, fewer incarcerations, a lower tendency to spend free time alone, and feeling less troubled by psychological problems.

DISCUSSION

The two major goals of the study were to assess differential effectiveness of the treatment interventions and to explore various predictors of successful outcomes. Contrary to expectations, there were virtually no differences among groups on outcomes, yet all groups showed dramatic improvements over time.

Pre-Post Differences

Concerning why there appeared to be such strong effects over time, there are several possible explanations. First, clients were recruited into the study at a point where they were entering a homeless shelter which for many was a low point in their lives. Given the cyclical nature of addiction where drug users abuse drugs, attempt to stay "clean" and then relapse, obtaining a sample of drug users at their lowest point may make it difficult not to show some improvement over the course of a year. This is akin to a regression to the mean effect when clients are selected at an extreme point in their functioning.

A second possibility is that clients exaggerated their drug usage at intake in order to make sure that they would receive services or because they believed that was what the intake workers wanted to hear; and then exaggerated their progress so as to please researchers at the follow-up point. Some prior research seems to indicate that self-reports of drinking and other drug use tend to be biased toward *underreporting* at baseline when clients are still using or are experiencing withdrawal,[7-9] with more accurate reporting occurring later when clients have been involved in treatment.[10-12] If this is true for the present study, then we would expect to find a bias toward finding a smaller difference between baseline and follow-up. Given the dramatic declines in drug use and increased employment and residential stability, this does not seem to be the case. A third possibility is a rather obvious one–that services may have a positive impact on clients, particularly when they are provided to clients who are at a low point in their lives. Thus, the provision of services to clients who are especially distressed may produce particularly strong positive effects.

Lack of Between Group Differences

Given the substantial baseline to follow-up impacts, the question remains as to why there were no differential effects among treatment groups. One possible explanation is that the comparison group was not a true control group in the traditional sense of a non-treatment group. Although case loads were quite high for Group 3 case managers, the clients were able to obtain many more services, either through case managers or on their own, than we had initially anticipated. In fact, there were virtually no differences in the amount or types of services received in the prior 60 days across groups at the discharge and follow-up assessment points (see Shipley et al.[5] for more detail on these analyses).

Another possible explanation, which is difficult to evaluate, concerns a possible "Hawthorne Effect" that may have been caused by the act of conducting the study. Based on our observations and interviews with service providers from Group 3, there did appear to be an enhanced level of service delivery compared to what we had perceived prior to initiating the project. Also, a decline in the total number of beds in the shelter during the course of the study reduced the size of the active caseloads of the Group 3 case managers, thus perhaps enhancing their effectiveness (making Group 3 case management somewhat more "intensive"). All of these possible explanations may have been operating simultaneously which, in combination, might have greatly increased the likelihood of finding no differences in treatment effectiveness across groups.

Predictions of Treatment Success

Fewer days of recent cocaine use at baseline predicted fewer days of use at follow-up; similarly, greater employment and more stable housing at baseline predicted greater employment and stable housing at follow-up. Conversely, criminal history was significantly related to poorer outcomes for substance use and stable housing at follow-up. Clients with a more extensive history of treatment tended to show greater substance use at follow-up. This latter finding was contrary to expectations since some studies have shown that clients with greater prior treatment experience tend to have better outcomes.[13,14] It may be that treatment exposure acted as a proxy for chronicity since it was also shown that the amount of prior use was a significant predictor of increased use at follow-up. Thus, in general, clients with more severe substance abuse histories, both in terms of recent and lifetime use, appeared to have poorer outcomes, with recent use seeming to be somewhat more predictive of subsequent outcomes than lifetime use variables. Demographic variables did not predict outcomes well.

Variables dealing with interpersonal relationships appeared to be associated with success. This may suggest that clients who are heavier users may have fewer social supports, be more socially isolated, and may be expected to do worse in treatment. How social isolation relates to homelessness and substance abuse is somewhat unclear–whether it is because of their homelessness and substance use that they are isolated, or whether these conditions are somehow a consequence of social isolation. However, the more socially isolated, the worse the outcomes.

In sum, clients who presented a less chronic and extreme history of substance use, homelessness, criminal activity, and social isolation, no matter what their age or educational level, tended to be able to better overcome their addiction and homeless state.

Implications

The results of our study point to several implications. First, although there was no differential effectiveness across treatment modalities, the substantial improvement manifested by the entire sample over time may suggest that services make a difference. Although it is probable that some of the improvement may be attributable to recruiting clients at an extreme point in their functioning as mentioned above, nearly all clients received some services (particularly involvement in 12-step groups) and it is likely that providing some services may make a difference for these men. Some of this improvement may be related to self-motivation as well as to readiness for treatment. Those who were not ready to commit to treatment often dropped out. Also, interviews with clients who were successful revealed the importance of self-motivation.[15] Both outcome research on substance abuse treatment and initial clinical assessments should focus on motivation for treatment as an important baseline measurement.[16] Treatment providers should explore ways of enhancing client motivation and ways of maintaining engagement to programs with clients who lack a strong commitment to treatment. Social support and motivation for treatment probably interact considerably, but more research needs to be done on the specific ways that these influence treatment outcomes.

In addition, our results particularly point to the importance of interpersonal relationships. Those who were more isolated tended to be less successful, and clients who have been successful in treatment frequently mention the importance of support from staff, other clients, friends and relatives as being critical for their recovery. The implication of this is that in developing effective programs for homeless substance abusers, an array of other institutions can and should be called upon to help reintegrate the homeless into society. Self-help groups have been an important support in these areas, but there are other sources within the typical community which can be called upon to reinforce the process. The emphasis should be on re-integrating clients with their communities to enhance social support and reduce isolation.

Finally, it was evident that the success of treatment is particularly challenged by clients who have more chronic problems relative to substance abuse. Differentiations may need to be made during initial intake assessments of clients who may be particularly difficult to treat on the basis of greater lifetime and recent substance use patterns. These clients should be targeted for special programmatic initiatives because of their poor prognosis.

REFERENCES

1. Conrad KJ, Hultman CI, Lyons JS, eds. Treatment of the chemically dependent homeless: Theory and implementation in fourteen American projects. New York: Haworth Press, 1993.

2. McLellan AT, Luborsky L, Cacciola J, McGahan P, O'Brien CP. Guide to the Addiction Severity Index: Background, administration, and field testing results. Washington, D.C.: National Institute on Drug Abuse, 1988.

3. Barrow SM, Hellman F, Lovell AM, Plapinger JD, Robinson CR, Struening EL. Personal History Form. Community Support Systems Evaluation Program, Epidemiology of Mental Disorders Research Department. New York: New York State Psychiatric Institute, 1985.

4. Attkisson CC, Zwick R. The Client Satisfaction Questionnaire, psychometric properties and correlations with service utilization and psychotherapy outcome. Evaluation and Program Planning 1982; 5:233-237.

5. Shipley TE, Stahler GJ, Bartelt D, Shandler I, and Goss E. Assessing alternative treatment methods for homeless polydrug addicted men: The Philadelphia Homeless Project. Final technical report to the National Institute of Alcohol Abuse and Alcoholism on Cooperative Agreement Grant 1 U01 AA08802. Philadelphia: Temple University and the Diagnostic and Rehabilitation Center, 1994.

6. Stahler GJ, Shipley TE, Bartelt D, Westcott D, Griffith E, Shandler I. Retention issues in treating homeless polydrug users. Alcoholism Treatment Quarterly 1993; 10:201-215.

7. Orwin RG, Sonnefeld LJ, Garrison-Mogren R, Smith NG. Pitfalls in evaluating the effectiveness of case management programs for homeless persons: Lessons from the NIAAA Community Demonstration Program. Eval Rev. 1994; 18: 153-207.

8. Skinner, HA. Assessing alcohol use by patients in treatment. In Smart RG, Cappell HD, Glaser FB, Israel Y, Kalant H, Popham RE, Schmidt W, Sellers EM, eds. Research advances in alcohol and drug problems, volume 8. New York: Plenum, 1984.

9. Sobell LC, Sobell MB. Effects of three interview factors on the validity of alcohol abusers' self-reports. Am J of Drug and Alcohol Abuse 1981; 8: 225-237.

10. Aiken LS, West SG. Invalidity of true experiments: Self-report pretest biases. Eval Rev. 1990; 14:374-390.

11. Hesselbrock M, Babor TF, Hesselbrock V, Meyer RE, Workman K. Never believe an alcoholic?: On the validity of self-report measures of alcohol dependence and related constructs. Int'l J of the Addictions 1983; 1 8:593-609.

12. Polich JM. The validity of self-reports in alcoholism research. Addictive Behaviors 1982; 7:123-132.

13. Federer MB, McHenry PC, Howard L. Factors related to the treatment of drug addicts enrolled in a residential rehabilitation facility. Advances in Alcohol and Substance Abuse 1986; 5:85-97.

14. Means LB, Small M, Capone DM, Capone TJ, Condren R, Peterson M, Hayward B. Client demographics and outcome in outpatient cocaine treatment. Intl J of the Addictions 1989; 24:765-783.

15. Stahler GJ, Cohen E, Greene MA, Shipley TE, Bartelt D. A qualitative study of treatment success among homeless crack addicted men: Definitions and attributions. Contemp Drug Probs, 1995; 22: in press.

16. DeLeon G, and Jainchill N. Circumstances, motivation, readiness, and suitability as correlates of tenure in treatment. J of Psychoactive Drugs 1986; 18: 203-208.

Factors That Interact with Treatment to Predict Outcomes in Substance Abuse Programs for the Homeless

James D. Wright, PhD
Joel A. Devine, PhD

SUMMARY. This paper reviews the main treatment effects observed in the New Orleans Homeless Substance Abusers Project and then analyzes and discusses factors that appear to interact with treatment to produce successful treatment outcomes. Outcomes are assessed for alcohol and drug use, housing stability, and employment. Results show marginally significant positive effects for long-term treatment, but only for clients retained in treatment for more than about three months. Holding treatment variables constant, client characteristics that predict successful treatment outcomes include gender, education, age, psychiatric morbidity, drug of choice, attendance at AA/NA meetings, and prior treatment histories. Some of these same factors also predict success among controls. The significance, sign, and magnitude of these effects, however, varies depending on which

James D. Wright and Joel A. Devine are affiliated with the Department of Sociology, Tulane University, New Orleans, LA.

Address correspondenc to James D. Wright, Department of Sociology, 220 Newcomb Hall, Tulane University, New Orleans, LA 70118.

Research reported here was supported by a research demonstration grant from the National Institute of Alcohol Abuse and Alcoholism, who bears no responsibility for the analyses or conclusions.

[Haworth co-indexing entry note]: "Factors that Interact with Treatment to Predict Outcomes in Substance Abuse Programs for the Homeless." Wright, James D., and Joel A. Devine. Co-published simultaneously in the *Journal of Addictive Diseases* (The Haworth Medical Press, an imprint of The Haworth Press, Inc.) Vol. 14, No. 4, 1995, pp. 169-181; and: *The Effectiveness of Social Interventions for Homeless Substance Abusers* (ed: Gerald J. Stahler) The Haworth Medical Press, an imprint of The Haworth Press, Inc., 1995, pp. 169-181. Single or multiple copies of this article are available from The Haworth Document Delivery Service [1-800-342-9678; 9:00 a.m. - 5:00 p.m. (EST)].

169

specific outcome one analyzes. Thus, variation in treatment effectiveness *is* associated with entering conditions, as the literature suggests, but which entering conditions matter most depends on which specific outcome one examines. *[Article copies available from The Haworth Document Delivery Service: 1-800-342-9678.]*

INTRODUCTION

The New Orleans Homeless Substance Abusers Program (NOHSAP) was a residentially-based adult resocialization project for homeless alcohol and drug abusers in the New Orleans area. Like all large cities with high poverty rates, New Orleans has a large homeless population estimated at approximately 8,000 persons. The New Orleans Task Force on Hunger and Homelessness estimates that nearly three-quarters of the city's homeless abuse alcohol, and that more than half abuse other drugs, much higher rates of substance abuse than reported for the national homeless population.[1] Moreover, there are very few programs for indigent alcohol and drug-abusive people in the city. At its peak capacity, NOHSAP alone accounted for more than a tenth of the total treatment options accessible to the New Orleans homeless.

PROGRAM PHILOSOPHY AND INTERVENTIONS

NOHSAP was designed to achieve four principal goals: (1) a drug- and alcohol-free existence; (2) residential stability; (3) economic independence; and (4) a reduction in family estrangement and an increase in general social functioning. (Additional details on program philosophy and implementation have been published elsewhere.[2]) The program was a three-phase intervention: Social or Family Detoxification (the control condition), Transitional Care (TC: the short-term treatment condition), and Extended Care/Independent Living (ECIL: the long-term treatment condition).

- Detox was a 7-day program of sobering up, introduction to AA and NA principles, twice-daily group meetings, some counselling, and limited assessment and case management. Clients judged *not* motivated or *not* suitable for further treatment by the clinical staff (i.e., were perceived as uncommitted to working their program and/or deemed to be non-compliant) were discharged and released to the streets. Clients deemed suitable for further treatment went into a pool of eligibles from which they were either randomized into treatment or released back to the streets. Social detox was a state-funded program for single individuals; family detox was a grant-funded program mainly for women with children. Otherwise, both programs were similar in design and intent.

- TC consisted of a 21-day program involving more extensive assessment and case management, twice-daily group meetings, placement in an off-campus alcohol or drug group, and general reinforcement of positive steps taken during detox. Clients successfully completing TC became eligible for ECIL.
- ECIL was a 12-month program that continued the interventions and strategies begun during TC while also providing GED services, job training, and job placement. Movement from TC to ECIL was determined by the same randomization process governing earlier entry into TC: clinical staff determined client suitability for further treatment; from this pool of eligibles, clients were either randomized into ECIL or released.

DESCRIPTION OF CLIENT POPULATION

Clients were overwhelmingly African-American (82.2%), relatively young (mean age = 34), and predominantly male (75%). Most had some work history and a few job skills, but as a whole they were ill-prepared for employment in the post-industrial economy. Just under half of the clients (48%) did not complete high school, and employment histories tended to be irregular and discontinuous. Monthly income from employment averaged $284 for the men and $70 for the women, but on average, the largest share of income (during the month prior to program entry) was derived from various illegal activities. A slight majority (52.5%) were poly-substance abusive; about half (47.6%) had alcohol problems; most (84.9%) were crack addicts; small proportions abused heroin and other illicit drugs. A quarter (26.9%) of the respondents had had previous treatment for their alcohol problems, and more than half (54.0%) had prior drug treatment histories as well.

Clients of both genders were estranged from family. The literature on familial disaffiliation among the adult homeless often intimates that most spent their early years within a stable home environment, that their ties to that environment were later disrupted, and that as a consequence of that disruption, they ended up on the streets. The actual pattern observed in these data is that the processes of disaffiliation and estrangement often stretch back to early childhood and that the "final break" that puts someone on the streets is less a disruption in an otherwise placid family situation than the culmination of a life-long process.[3]

Forty-five percent of the entering clients were recently homeless for the first time, 23% were episodically homeless (multiple prior episodes of homelessness punctuated by variable periods of stable housing), and the remaining 32% were identified as chronically homeless (homeless more or less continuously since the first onset of homelessness). The recently homeless were disproportionately women. Crack addicts were over-represented among the recently homeless; alcoholics were over-represented among the episodic and chronic groups.

In sum, NOHSAP clients were poor, unemployed, estranged from family, homeless, and chemically addicted–in a word, the urban underclass.[4] They also suffered from degraded physical and mental health and were frequently in trouble with the law–factors that complicate treatment in numerous ways. On the whole, the NOHSAP population differed little in background and social characteristics from urban homeless populations described in any number of prior studies.[5-6]

SAMPLE SIZES, RANDOMIZATION, AND RESEARCH ATTRITION

NOHSAP began seeing clients in February 1991. Over the next fourteen months, 670 clients were baselined into the study. Of these, 505 (75.4%) were "controls" (who received seven days of detoxification and were released back to the community) while 165 (24.6%) entered one or both of the treatment conditions (as below). Six-month follow-up interviews were obtained on 620 (92.5%) clients.[7] Outcome analyses are based on these 620 clients for whom six-month follow-up data are available.

Although assignment to treatment and control conditions was theoretically random, random assignment was seriously compromised in the field implementation.[8] Nonetheless, with a single notable (and statistically controllable) exception–gender–the essential equivalence of the treatment and control groups was maintained. Women were far more likely to be placed in TC and ECIL than men. However, once this factor is taken into account, the non-equivalences between treatment and control groups vanish on nearly all other variables. To account for this selection bias, gender is held constant in all analyses.

Net attrition due to failure to follow up clients amounted to only about 7% of the baselined sample and was virtually identical in both treatment and control groups. Located and unlocated clients are not statistically distinguishable on the vast majority of variables examined. Thus, no statistical adjustments are necessary to account for differential attrition from treatment and control conditions.

RESULTS: MAIN EFFECTS OF TREATMENT

The following summarizes the main effects observed in the analysis of NOHSAP six-month outcome data; the final report on the project[9] gives a more complete description of the results.

Sobriety: Concerning relapse to alcohol, all treatment groups did better than controls, but the differences were modest except for ECIL clients completing more than the median number of treatment days (see Treatment Attrition). Concerning relapse to other drugs, the data do not show even marginally significant treatment effects, although long-term ECIL clients did slightly better than other groups on most indicators. We conclude that any treatment beyond detoxification conferred marginally positive benefits in the area of sobriety and relapse, that these benefits were most pronounced for long-term ECIL clients, but that the treatment benefits were stronger for relapse to alcohol than for relapse to other drugs.

Other Programmatic Goals: Success in achieving the project's secondary goals was also spotty. Long-term ECIL clients tended to do better in the areas of housing, employment, and income than others, but the effects were rarely large and only occasionally significant. All NOHSAP treatments appear to have conferred some employment benefits for women; long-term ECIL stays conferred significantly strong employment and income benefits for both men and women. There is also fairly consistent evidence that long-term ECIL stays were helpful in avoiding subsequent spells of homelessness but did not result in fewer days of homelessness for those who did experience homeless episodes. Long-term ECIL clients were also much more successful in finding their own places to stay (as opposed to living with others or concocting other housing arrangements). All indicators of post-treatment housing status therefore suggest that long-term ECIL clients did marginally to significantly better than controls, but TC clients and short-term ECIL clients did not.

Concerning tertiary outcomes such as family and social relationships, service utilization, physical health, emotional well-being, and legal problems, the data revealed no consistent or significant treatment effects.

Treatment Attrition: Although ECIL was intended as a 12-month program, very few clients actually completed the full twelve months; in fact, the average length of stay for clients placed in ECIL was only 166 days (or about four months post-TC). In general, ECIL clients completing less than the average length of stay were indistinguishable from TC-only clients on practically all outcomes, from which we infer that interventions of 2-5 months duration generally do not confer benefits over and beyond those conferred in a one-month intervention. Stays in excess of the average length of stay, on the other hand, were consistently related to positive outcomes.

As a matter of fact, retention in treatment is the single strongest predictor of success in treatment regardless of treatment modality or the type of client population served[10-13] and in this NOHSAP was certainly no exception.

Detailed analyses of retention in treatment produced only marginally significant or interesting results. Given the strong initial selection bias in favor of women, we wondered whether gender would predict retention in treatment as well. It did not. Among a large number of other demographic variables we examined, only race emerged as a marginally significant predictor; blacks averaged 29 *more* days in treatment than whites. Other background variables such as age, gender, religion and the like were always insignificant regardless of the specific models being tested. Likewise, among a long list of variables indexing clients' homelessness status and history, the only marginally significant predictor of retention in treatment was whether the client was first-time (as opposed to episodic or chronic) homeless. Four variables reflecting clients' alcohol and drug histories proved to be significant (or marginally significant) predictors of retention in treatment. Clients who mentioned alcohol as either their first or second substance problem averaged 26 *more* days in treatment than clients who did not; in contrast, clients who mentioned crack cocaine as either their first or second substance problem averaged 43 *fewer* days in treatment than those who did not; on the other hand, the *severity* of a client's alcohol problem was *negatively* related to retention in treatment. Finally, clients with previous alcohol or drug treatment histories averaged 18 *fewer* days in treatment than clients for whom NOHSAP was their first treatment experience.

These analyses of retention in treatment are more interesting for what they do not show than for what they do. Among the several ASI composite scores, only the alcohol variable predicted retention in treatment; the other composites were insignificant in all analyses. We take this as fairly persuasive evidence that the clinical staff did *not* attempt to deal with the most troubled or problematic clients by finding reasons to terminate their treatment. Alcohol and drug use in the previous thirty days or years of alcohol and drug use over the lifetime were also insignificant in most analyses. Various indicators of clients' psychiatric status (severity of psychological problems, psychiatric hospitalizations, etc.) were also insignificant. Thus, with the partial exception of the variables already mentioned, we conclude that *nothing* systematically predicts retention in treatment. In one sense, this is an encouraging result; it shows that clinical staff did not systematically terminate (or prematurely shorten treatment of) certain classes of clients even where it might have been advantageous to do so. On the other hand, these findings leave unexplained a rather curious anomaly, namely, that so many ECIL clients left the program well in advance of their allotted twelve (or thirteen) months.

Our speculation (consistent with what is known about addiction) is that while nearly anyone could successfully cope with the thought of a week or even a month without alcohol and drugs, the looming possibility of an entire *year* clean and sober (not to say a lifetime) proved to be more than a little daunting to many. It is also plausible that many ECIL clients tired quickly of the restrictions on sexual relations or wished to reconnect with outside partners; many may have also balked at the many rules and regulations that dictated behavior within the NOHSAP facility. Finally, many clients seem to feel that they are "in control" after two or three months, that they can "handle" themselves on the outside, that they are "ready" for independence, and so they leave treatment only to find that the temptations of the outside world are overwhelming. Whatever the specific reasons, our difficulty in maintaining clients in treatment for much more than a few months suggests that homeless addicts often cannot be retained in treatment long enough for treatment to have significantly positive effects.

RESULTS: FACTORS THAT PREDICT SUCCESS IN TREATMENT

NOHSAP clients had highly variable backgrounds, familial and social circumstances, alcohol and drug histories, homelessness experiences, etc. How is variation in these characteristics related to success in treatment, independently of the effects of treatment itself?

Early research on drug and alcohol treatment was focused on the beguilingly simple question, "Does treatment work?" In the aggregate, treatment effects were typically shown to be small or non-existent, and of relatively short duration when they were found to exist at all.[10-13] Addiction disorder specialists soon recognized, however, that the conclusion of small or non-significant overall treatment effects overlooked a great deal of individual variation in response to treatment. Some clients, that is, showed dramatic improvement after treatment, many showed no change, and still others showed negative outcomes. And so the research question evolved from "Does treatment work?" to "With what kinds of clients is treatment most effective?" How, in short, do initial client characteristics condition responsiveness to drug and alcohol treatment?

Numerous client characteristics have been investigated in this connection, including drug of choice, client motivation, prior treatment histories, severity of psychiatric symptoms, race, and other factors.[14] McLellan et al.

TABLE 1. Basic Model.

	Outcome							
	Good Days		Substance Free Days		Days Housed		Days Working	
	b	p	b	p	b	p	b	p
Baseline Value	.257	.00	.146	.05	.118	.03	.388	.00
Treatment Days	.012	.03	.011	.26	.003	.60	.022	.01
Adjusted R^2 =	.08		.03		.02		.14	
N =	145		148		151		150	

showed that drug and alcohol treatment was most effective in clients with mild to moderate levels of entering psychopathology and generally ineffective in patients with more severe psychiatric impairments.[15] It has also been shown that highly-motivated clients respond better to all forms of treatment than unmotivated clients.

In order to examine the effects of initial client characteristics on responsiveness to NOHSAP treatment, we chose four outcome variables: the number of days (of the thirty prior to follow-up) that the client was substance free (used neither alcohol nor drugs), the number of days not homeless, the number of days the client worked for pay, and a summary measure of "total good days" (basically, the sum of the other outcome measures). The analysis focuses only on treatment clients (N = 152). To account for the main effects of treatment summarized above, each model includes total days in treatment among the regressors; the corresponding baseline value for each outcome variable is also included in all models.

We began with a "basic model" containing *only* the corresponding baseline values and days in treatment as regressors (Table 1). Baseline values significantly (defined as p < .10, given the small sample size) predict follow-up values in all cases; the coefficients for days working and total good days are particularly strong (i.e., clients who had more good days in the month before they entered treatment also had more good days in the month before follow-up). That said, the coefficients for total days in treatment are also always positive but only significant in the equations for days working and total good days. This is consistent with our general conclusion that NOHSAP had marginally positive outcomes in most areas but significantly positive outcomes only in some areas. Note finally that the largest share of the variation in outcome is independent of baseline values

TABLE 2. Basic Model, Demographic Characteristics, Psychopathology, Alcohol and Drug Histories, Prior Treatment, First-Time Homeless, Family and Social Problems, Attendance at AA/NA Meetings.

	Outcome							
	Good Days		Substance Free Days		Days Housed		Days Working	
	b	p	b	p	b	p	b	p
Baseline Value	.237	.00	.020	.77	.093	.08	.303	.00
Treatment Days	.011	.02	.010	.21	.005	.42	.019	.01
Gender	-2.301	.00	---	NS	2.202	.06	-4.460	.00
Education	.637	.00	.611	.07	.766	.00	.858	.01
Age	---	NS	-.171	.11	-.172	.03	---	NS
Kids	---	NS	---	NS	-2.268	.08	---	NS
ASI Psychiatric Composite Score	---	NS	---	NS	---	NS	-6.800	.05
Crack	-6.750	.00	---	NS	---	NS	-13.852	.00
ASI Alcohol Composite Score	---	NS	-5.447	.04	---	NS	---	NS
Prior Treatment	-.307	.01	---	NS	---	NS	-.196	.02
1st-time Homles	---	NS	--	NS	-1.787	.10	---	NS
ASI Fam/Social Composite Score	2.618	.07	5.376	.03	---	NS	---	NS
Attend AA/NA	3.092	.00	7.984	.00	---	NS	---	NS
Adjusted R^2 =	.38		.34		.13		.32	
N =	137		139		151		146	

and days in treatment; the R^2 values are generally low, ranging from 2% (days housed) to 14% (days paid for working).

Holding baseline values and days in treatment constant, we then explored the residual effects of a number of social, demographic, treatment history, psychiatric, and other variables on treatment outcomes. Variables were entered in classes and a best-fitting model was derived in step-wise fashion, with significant predictors from each step being carried over into the next step. Many of the variables we explored were insignificant and are therefore dropped from further consideration (e.g., race). Table 2 summarizes the "best-fitting" model; the following text describes the results obtained in each intervening step.

In the step adding socio-demographic variables, the baseline values and days in treatment measures continued to operate as before (in the basic model). In addition, the effect for education is strong, positive, and generally significant; treatment clients with a high school education or better responded more positively across the board. (As a matter of fact, *control* clients with more education also showed consistently better outcomes than less educated controls.) The effects of gender are mixed but, net of other variables, women are more likely than men to obtain housing, less likely than men to obtain employment, and just as likely as men to relapse. Age and having one's children with them in treatment also had a *negative* impact on later housing status (though the latter was only marginally significant). Finally, adding socio-demographic variables to the models substantially increased the explained variance; the R^2 values range from 12% to 25%, higher in every case than the values for the basic equations.

We next explored a set of variables concerning early childhood and adolescent experiences (e.g., variables indexing when the client first started drinking, when he or she first tried hard drugs, and a composite index of "family of origin dysfunctionality" based on familial alcohol, drug, or psychiatric problems, childhood abuse, time spent in foster care, etc.). However, none of these variables proved significant in any equation.

As noted above, McLellan[14-15] has reported in a number of studies that entering mental health status is an important conditioner of effectiveness of treatment. While a variable indexing the number of prior psychiatric hospitalizations was not significant in any equation, we did find that the ASI composite score for psychological and emotional problems was significantly and negatively related to days paid for working. This suggests that more emotionally troubled clients experienced more employment difficulties than less troubled clients but showed neither better nor worse performance on other outcomes. Thus, contrary to findings from McLellan and associates, we do not find that treatment works better for those with mild to non-existent psychiatric disturbance, except in the area of employment.

We next tested a set of variables representing clients' alcohol and drug histories. The pattern of the results was mixed. Clients with a crack problem had significantly fewer days paid for working and significantly fewer total good days, but the variable was not significant in the other two equations. Likewise, clients with higher ASI *alcohol* problem composite scores had significantly fewer substance-free days. No other variable was significant in any equation. We conclude that, while there is some evidence that clients with less severe alcohol and drug problems to begin with respond somewhat better to treatment, the effects are not nearly as strong or as consistent across variables as one might expect. With a few exceptions, adding these variables to the models also leaves the other effects largely intact; with these variables included, the explanatory power of the models is also noticeably enhanced.

Two other variables were tested in the next step, both plausibly related to treatment effectiveness. The first is a baseline measure of AA-style "spirituality," which we expected to emerge as a significant predictor of responsiveness to treatment. The variable was insignificant in all equations. Another variable of interest is prior treatment history. In brief, we expected this variable to be *positively* related to outcomes. Sobriety, like drunkenness, is learned behavior and like any other learned behavior, takes some practice before one gets it right. In fact, prior treatment histories were significant predictors of both days paid for working and total good days, but the effect was *negative* in both cases.

As a final step, we also explored a number of variables representing clients' homelessness histories, the ASI composite indicators not yet included in the models, and a number of other variables suggested in the treatment outcome literature.[10-15] Among variables reflecting homelessness histories, only a dummy variable for first-time homeless was significant, and that only in the equation predicting days in housing (where the effect was negative). Among the remaining ASI composite scores, only that reflecting family and social relationship problems was significant. Clients with higher scores on the variable (i.e, with *more* serious problems) had *more* substance-free days and *more* total good days than clients with lower scores. This effect suggests that estrangement from families is *positively* functional for recovery from alcohol and drug disorders, a very plausible finding given the high level of dysfunctionality characterizing the families of many of these clients. The other ASI composite scores (reflecting problems with physical health, employment, and legal matters) were insignificant in all equations.

Among the other variables considered, only one emerged as a significant predictor in several equations: whether the client was attending AA or NA meetings. Attendance at AA/NA meetings was fairly strongly and positively related to the number of substance-free days and the total number of good days. We are not certain how to interpret this effect; we suspect that the variable is a proxy for the client's initial level of motivation. That is, clients with sufficient initial motivation to attend AA or NA meetings once released from treatment do better than other clients. Other analyses also suggested, however, that NOHSAP treatment itself had a marked, positive effect on post-release AA/NA attendance; moreover, the treatment coefficients are largely independent of AA/NA attendance in the final model (see Table 2). (Thus, AA/NA attendance is an exogenous, not intervening, variable conditioning outcomes.) As it happens, attendance at AA and NA meetings is also related to substance-free days and total good days among *controls*.

The final models are shown in Table 2. As models in the social sciences go, these models are actually rather good. In a few cases, variables that were significant become insignificant in the final models, but most of the effects are robust in the face of successive respecifications (both surprising and encouraging given the sample sizes and the large number of factors retained in each model). It is especially encouraging to note that the initially significant coefficients for days in treatment remain significant even with all other variables held constant; thus, the previously discussed positive treatment effects are apparently *not* artifacts of uncontrolled differences in initial conditions. Finally, with the exception of the model predicting days in housing, the R^2 values are respectably high, explaining a third or more of the variation in treatment outcomes.

CONCLUSION

Concerning the main effects of treatment, the principal conclusion is that NOHSAP conferred marginally to strongly positive benefits for clients who were retained in treatment for more than a few months, but that most clients could not be so retained; stays of less than a few months conferred no benefits beyond those associated with TC. In fact, the coefficients for TC were themselves rarely significant, implying that the TC program was, at best, only a marginal improvement over seven days of detoxification.

Analyses of the factors that predict treatment outcomes shows that with one exception (days substance-free), baseline values are positive and significant predictors of follow-up values. Days in treatment are positively associated with all outcomes but significantly related only to days paid for working and total good days. Education is significantly and positively related to all outcomes. Factors predicting other outcomes vary depending on the outcome in question. Thus, variation in treatment effectiveness *is* systematically associated with entering conditions, as the literature suggests, but *which entering conditions matter most depends on which outcome one examines.* Other than baseline values and client's education, nothing systematically predicts outcomes across the board.

The consistently positive effect of education is surprising and hitherto unnoted in the treatment literature. Education proved more important than entering problem severity, drug of choice, prior treatment history, and most other variables in predicting outcomes. Two hypotheses might be entertained as an explanation for the effect. First, NOHSAP was mainly a cognitive and didactic intervention; to the extent that education is a proxy for cognitive skill, one would expect the treatment to "take" more firmly among those with higher skills. A second possibility is that education is a proxy for life chances; the better educated, that is, have greater human capital that can be used to negotiate recovery and likewise would have more to gain (presumably) by staying clean and sober. We are unable to choose between these possibilities given the data in hand, but the effect is sufficiently consistent and strong to make it worth looking for in other contexts and populations.

REFERENCES

1. Wright JD, Weber E. Homelessness and health. Washington, DC: McGraw Hill, 1987.

2. Wright JD, Devine JA, Eddington N. The New Orleans homeless substance abusers program. Alcoholism Treatment Quarterly 1993; 10 (3-4): 51-64.

3. Wright JD, Devine JA. Family backgrounds and the substance-abusive homeless: the New Orleans experience. The Community Psychologist 1993; 26:35-37.

4. Devine JA, Wright JD. The greatest of evils: urban poverty and the American underclass. Hawthorne, NY: Aldine de Gruyter, 1993.

5. Wright JD. Address unknown: the homeless in America. Hawthorne, New York: Aldine de Gruyter, 1989.

6. Rossi PH. Down and out in America. Chicago: University of Chicago Press, 1990.

7. Wright JD, Allen TL, Devine JA. Tracking non-traditional populations in longitudinal surveys. Evaluation and Program Planning 1995; in press.

8. Devine JA, Wright JD, Joyner LM. Issues in implementing a randomized experiment in a field settings. New Directions for Program Evaluation, 1994; 63:27-40.

9. Wright JD, Devine JA, Joyner LM. The least of mine: the New Orleans homeless substance abusers project final report. Final report to the National Institute of Alcohol Abuse and Alcoholism, Washington, DC, 1993.

10. Gerstein DR, Harwood HJ (eds). Treating drug problems. Volume I. Washington, DC: National Academy Press, 1990.

11. Joe GW, Singh BK, Garland J, Lehman W, Sells SB, Seder P. Retention in outpatient drug-free treatment clinics. Addictive Behaviors 1983; 8:219-234.

12. Joe GW, Simpson DD, Hubbard RL. Treatment predictors of tenure in methadone maintenance. Journal of Substance Abuse 1991; 3: 73-84.

13. Wright JD, Devine JA. Drugs as a social problem. New York: Harper Collins, 1994.

14. McLellan AT. Patient characteristics associated with outcome. In Cooper, Altman, Brown and Czechowicz (eds), Research on the treatment of narcotic addiction: state of the art. Washington, DC: US Government Printing Office, 1983.

15. McLellan AT, Luborsky L, Woody GE, O'Brien CP, Druley KA. Predicting response to alcohol and drug abuse treatments. Archives of General Psychiatry 1983; 40:620-625.

SELECTIVE GUIDE TO CURRENT REFERENCE SOURCES ON TOPICS DISCUSSED IN THIS ISSUE

Social Interventions for Homeless Substance Abusers

Lynn Kasner Morgan, MLS

Each issue of *Journal of Addictive Diseases* features a section offering suggestions on where to look for further information on included topics. The intent is to guide readers to selective substantive sources of current information on the effectiveness of social interventions for homeless substance abusers.

Some published reference works utilize designated terminology (controlled vocabularies) which must be used to find material on topics of

Lynn Kasner Morgan is Assistant Professor of Medical Education, Assistant Dean for Information Resources and Systems, and Director of the Gustave L. and Janet W. Levy Library of the Mount Sinai Medical Center, Inc., One Gustave L., Levy Place, New York, NY 10029-6574.

[Haworth co-indexing entry note]: "Selective Guide to Current Reference Sources on Topics Discussed in this Issue: Social Interventions for Homeless Substance Abusers." Morgan, Lynn Kasner. Co-published simultaneously in the *Journal of Addictive Diseases* (The Haworth Medical Press, an imprint of The Haworth Press, Inc.) Vol. 14, No. 4, 1995, pp. 183-195; and: *The Effectiveness of Social Interventions for Homeless Substance Abusers* (ed: Gerald J. Stahler) The Haworth Medical Press, an imprint of The Haworth Press, Inc., 1995, pp. 183-195. Single or multiple copies of this article are available from The Haworth Document Delivery Service [1-800-342-9678; 9:00 a.m. - 5:00 p.m. (EST)].

interest. For these, a sample of available search terms has been indicated to assist the reader in accessing appropriate sources for his/her purposes. Other reference tools use keywords or free text terms from the title of the document, the abstract, and the name of any responsible agency or conference. In searching using keywords, be sure to look under all possible synonyms to retrieve the concept in question.

An asterisk (*) appearing before a published source indicates that all or part of that source is in machine-readable form and can be accessed through an online database search. Database searching is recommended for retrieving sources of information that coordinate multiple variables, concepts, or subject areas. Most health sciences libraries offer database services which can include mediated online searching, access to locally mounted datafiles, front-end software packages, and CD-ROM technology. Searching can also be done from one's office or home with subscriptions to database service vendors and microcomputers equipped with modems.

Interactive electronic communications systems, such as electronic mail, discussion groups, bulletin boards, and receiving and transferring files are available through the Internet, which offers timely and global information resources in all disciplines, including the health sciences. Some groups which might be of interest are: ALCOHOL (ALCOHOL@LMUACAD), DRUG ABUSE (DRUGABUS@UMAB), 12STEP@TRWRB.DSD.COM and ADDICTION MEDICINE (MAJORDOMO@AVOCADO.PC.HELSIN-KI.FI). There are also many sites with World Wide Web pages which can be reached by individuals with a Web browser such as Mosaic or Netscape. A suggested starting point is http://www.yahoo.com/health.

Readers are encouraged to consult their librarians for further assistance before undertaking research on a topic.

Suggestions regarding the content and organization of this section are welcome and should be sent to the author.

1. INDEXING AND ABSTRACTING SOURCES

Place of publication, publisher, start date, frequency of publication, and brief descriptions are noted.

*Biological Abstracts (1926-) and Biological Abstracts/RRM (v.18, 1980-). Philadelphia, BioSciences Information Service, semimonthly. Reports on worldwide research in the life sciences.

See: Concept headings for abstracts, such as behavioral biology, pharmacology, psychiatry, public health, and toxicology sections.

See: Keyword-in-context subject index.

Chemical Abstracts. Columbus, Ohio, American Chemical Society, 1907- , weekly. A key to the world's literature of chemistry and chemical engineering, including serial publications, proceedings and edited collections, technical reports, dissertations, new book and audiovisual materials announcements, and patent documents.

See: *Index Guide* for cross-referencing and indexing policies.

See: *General Subject Index* terms, such as drug dependence, drug-drug interactions, drug tolerance, opioids.

See: Keyword subject indexes.

Dissertation Abstracts International. Section A. The Humanities and Social Sciences and Section B. The Sciences and Engineering. Ann Arbor, Mich., University Microfilms, v.30, 1969/70- , monthly. Includes author-prepared abstracts of doctoral dissertations from 500 participating institutions throughout North America and the world. A separate section contains European dissertations.

See: Keyword subject index.

Excerpta Medica. Amsterdam, The Netherlands, Excerpta Medica Foundation, 1947- , 42 subject sections. A major abstracting service covering more than 4,300 biomedical journals. The abstracts, including English summaries for non-English-language articles, appear in one or more of the published subject sections, excluding Section 38, *Adverse Reactions Titles,* which is an index only. Each of the sections has a comprehensive subject index. Since 1978 all the *Excerpta Medica* sections have been available for computer searching in the integrated online file, EMBASE. Particularly relevant to the topics in this issue are Section 40, *Drug Dependence, Alcohol Abuse and Alcoholism;* and the sections that have addiction, alcoholism, or drug subdivisions: Section 30, *Clinical and Experimental Pharmacology*; Section 32, *Psychiatry*; and Section 17, *Public Health, Social Medicine and Epidemiology.*

Hospital Literature Index. Chicago, American Hospital Association, v. 13, 1957- , quarterly, with annual cumulatons. Published as the primary guide to literature on hospital and other health facility administration, including multi-institutional systems, health policy and planning, and administrative aspects of health care delivery.

> See: *MeSH* terms, such as alcoholism, homeless persons, outcome and process assessment, outcome assessment, residential facilities, social responsibility, substance abuse treatment centers.

Index Medicus (includes *Bibliography of Medical Reviews*). Bethesda, Md., National Library of Medicine, 1960- , monthly, with annual cumulations. Published as author and subject indexes to more than 3,000 journals in the biomedical sciences. Subject headings are based on the controlled vocabulary or thesaurus, *Medical Subject Headings (MeSH)*. Since 1966 it has been produced from the MEDLARS database, which provides more comprehensive retrieval, including keyword access and English-language abstracts, than its printed counterparts: *Index Medicus, International Nursing Index,* and *Index to Dental Literature.*

> See: *MeSH* terms, such as alcohol drinking; alcoholism; behavior, addictive; buprenorphine; cocaine; heroin; homeless persons; homeless youth; methadone; outcome assessment; patient dropouts; social responsibility; substance abuse; substance abuse treatment centers; substance dependence; substance withdrawal syndrome.

Index to Scientific Reviews. Philadelphia, Institute for Scientific Information, 1974- , semiannual.

> See: Permuterm keyword subject index.

> See: Citation index.

International Pharmaceutical Abstracts. Washington, D.C., American Society of Hospital Pharmacists, 1964- , semimonthly. A key to the world's literature of pharmacy.

> See: IPA subject terms, such as alcoholism, cocaine, controlled substances, dependence, drug abuse, drug withdrawal, methadone, opiates, outcomes, residential care facilities.

Psychological Abstracts. Washington, D.C., American Psychological Association, 1927- , monthly. A compilation of nonevaluative summaries of the world's literature in psychology and related disciplines.

> See: Index terms, such as addiction, alcoholism, alcohol rehabilitation, drug abuse, drug addiction, drug dependency, drug rehabilitation, drug usage, drug usage screening, drug withdrawal, heroin addiction, homeless, methadone, opiates, residential care institutions, social adjustment, social programs, social services, treatment outcomes.

Public Affairs Information Service Bulletin. New York, Public Affairs Information Service, v.55, 1969- , semimonthly. An index to library material in the field of public affairs and public policy published throughout the world.

> See: PAIS subject headings, such as alcoholism, cocaine, drug abuse, drug addicts, drugs, heroin, methadone, narcotics, opium, social policy, social problems, social service–work with alcoholics, social service–work with homeless persons.

Science Citation Index. Philadelphia, Institute for Scientific Information, 1961- , bimonthly.

> See: Permuterm keyword subject index.

> See: Citation index.

Social Planning/Policy & Development Abstracts. San Diego, Calif., Sociological Abstracts, Inc., v.6, 1984- , semiannual.

> See: Thesaurus and descriptors listed under *Sociological Abstracts.*

Social Work Abstracts. New York, National Association of Social Workers, v.13, 1977- , quarterly.

> See: Subject index.

Sociological Abstracts. San Diego, Calif., Sociological Abstracts, Inc., 1952- , 6 times per year. A collection of nonevaluative abstracts which reflect the world's serial literature in sociology and related disciplines.

> See: *Thesaurus of Sociological Indexing Terms.*

> See: Descriptors such as alcohol abuse, alcoholism, cocaine, drinking behavior, drug abuse, drug addiction, drug use, heroin, homelessness, mathadone maintenance, opiates, residential institutions, social services, substance abuse, treatment compliance, treatment methods, treatment outcomes, treatment programs.

Substance Abuse Index and Abstracts: A Guide to Drug, Alcohol and Tobacco Research. New York, Scientific DataLink, 1989- , annual with supplements. A multidisciplinary guide to the literature on psychoactive substance use and abuse, prevention, treatment and control.

> See: Subject index.

2. CURRENT AWARENESS PUBLICATIONS

Current Contents: Clinical Medicine. Philadelphia, Institute for Scientific Information, v.15, 1987- , weekly.

> See: Keyword index.

Current Contents: Life Sciences. Philadelphia, Institute for Scientific Information, v. 10, 1967-, weekly.

> See: Keyword index.

Current Contents: Social & Behavioral Sciences. Philadelphia, Institute for Scientific Information, v.6, 1974- , weekly.

See: Keyword index.

3. BOOKS

Andrews, Theodora. *A Bibliography of Drug Abuse, Including Alcohol and Tobacco.* Littleton, Colo., Libraries Unlimited, 1977-.

Andrews, Theodora. *Guide to the Literature of Pharmacy and the Pharmaceutical Sciences.* Littleton, Colo., Libraries Unlimited, 1986.

Medical and Health Care Books and Serials in Print: An Index to Literature in the Health Sciences. New York, R. R. Bowker Co., annual.

See: Library of Congress subject headings, such as alcoholism, cocaine, drug abuse, drugs, methadone, narcotic habit, rehabilitation.

Miller, Norman S., ed. *Comprehensive Handbook of Drug and Alcohol Addiction.* New York, Dekker, c1991.

National Library of Medicine Current Catalog. Bethesda, Md., National Library of Medicine, 1966-quarterly, with annual cumulations.

See: MeSH terms as noted in Section 1 under *Index Medicus.*

O'Brien, Robert [and others]. *The Encyclopedia of Drug Abuse.* 2nd ed. New York, Facts on File, c1992.

Stimmel, Barry [and others]. *The Facts About Drug Use: Coping with Drug Use in Your Family, at Work, in Your Community.* Mount Vernon, N.Y., Consumers' Union, c1991.

World Health Organization Catalogue: New Books. Geneva, World Health Organization, semiannual (supplements *World Health Organization Publications* and includes periodicals).

Substance Abuse: The Nation's Number One Health Problem. Key Indicators for Policy. Princeton, N.J., Robert Wood Johnson Foundation, 1993.

4. U.S. GOVERNMENT PUBLICATIONS

Alcohol and Other Drug Thesaurus: A Guide to Concepts and Terminology in Substance Abuse and Addiction (AOD Thesaurus). Rockville, Md., National Institute on Alcohol Abuse and Alcoholism, 1994.

*Monthly Catalog of United States Government Publications. Washington, D.C., U.S. Government Printing Office, 1895- , monthly.

See: Following agencies: Alcohol, Drug Abuse and Mental Health Administration; Center for Substance Abuse Prevention; Centers for Disease Control and Prevention; Food and Drug Administration; National Center for Health Statistics; National Institute of Mental Health; National Institute on Drug Abuse; National Institutes of Health.

See: Subject headings, derived chiefly from the Library of Congress, such as alcohol, alcoholics, alcoholism, ambulatory medical care, drug abuse, drug habit, drug interactions, drug utilization, drug dependence, drugs, narcotics, pharmacology, physician and patient.

See: Title index.

5. ONLINE BIBLIOGRAPHIC DATABASES

Only those databases which have no print counterparts are included in this section. Print sources which have online database equivalents are noted throughout this guide by the asterisk (*) which appears before the title. If you do not have direct access to these databases, consult your librarian for assistance.

ALCOHOL AND ALCOHOL PROBLEMS SCIENCE DATABASE: ETOH (National Institute on Alcohol Abuse and Alcoholism, Rockville, Md.).

Use: Keywords.

ALCOHOL INFORMATION FOR CLINICIANS AND EDUCATORS (Project Cork Institute, Dartmouth Medical School, Hanover, N.H.).

Use: Keywords.

ASI: AMERICAN STATISTICS INDEX (Congressional Information Services, Inc., Washington, D.C.).

Use: Keywords.

DRUG INFORMATION FULLTEXT (American Society of Hospital Pharmacists, Bethesda, Md.).

Use: Keywords.

DRUGINFO AND ALCOHOL USE AND ABUSE (Hazelden Foundation, Center City, Minn., and Drug Information Service Center, College of Pharmacy, University of Minnesota, Minneapolis, Minn.).

Use: Keywords.

FAMILY RESOURCES DATABASE (National Council on Family Relations and Inventory of Marriage and Family Literature Project, Minneapolis, Minn.).

Use: Keywords.

LEXIS (Mead Data Central, Inc., Dayton, Ohio).

Use: Keywords.

MAGAZINE INDEX (Information Access Co., Belmont, Calif.).

Use: Keywords.

MENTAL HEALTH ABSTRACTS (IFI/Plenum Data Co., Alexandria, Va.).

Use: Keywords.

NATIONAL NEWSPAPER INDEX (Information Access Co., Belmont, Calif.).

Use: Keywords.

NTIS (National Technical Information Service, U.S. Dept. of Commerce, Springfield, Va.).

Use: Keywords.

PSYCINFO (American Psychological Association, Washington, D.C.).

Use: Keywords.

QUICK FACTS (Cygnus Corporation, Alcohol Epidemiologic Data System, under contract with NIAAA, Washington, D.C.).

Use: Keywords.

WESTLAW (West Publishing Co., St. Paul, Minn.).

Use: Keywords.

6. HANDBOOKS, DIRECTORIES, GRANT SOURCES, ETC.

Annual Register of Grant Support. Wilmette, Ill., National Register Pub. Co., annual.

See: Internal medicine; medicine; pharmacology, psychiatry, psychology, mental health sections.

See: Subject index.

*Biomedical Index to PHS-Supported Research. Bethesda, Md., National Institutes of Health, Division of Research Grants, annual.

See: Subject index.

Database Directory. White Plains, N.Y., Knowledge Industry Publications in cooperation with the American Society for Information Science, annual.

See: Subject index.

Directory of Research Grants. Phoenix, Ariz., Oryx Press, annual.

See: Subject index terms, such as drug abuse.

Encyclopedia of Associations. Detroit, Gale Research Co., annual (occasional supplements between editions).

See: Subject index.

Foundation Directory. New York, The Foundation Center, biennial (updated between editions by Foundation Directory Supplement).

See: Index of foundations.

See: Index of foundations by state and city.

See: Index of donors, trustees, and administrators.

See: Index of fields of interest.

Health Hotlines: Toll-Free Numbers from DIRLINE. Bethesda, Md., National Library of Medicine, biennial.

Information Industry Directory. Detroit, Gale Research Co., annual.

Nolan, Kathleen Lopez. *Gale Directory of Databases.* Detroit, Gale Research, Inc., 1995.

Roper, Fred W. and Jo Anne Boorkman. *Introduction to Reference Sources in the Health Sciences.* 3rd ed. Chicago, Medical Library Association, c1994.

The SALIS Directory: Substance Abuse Librarians and Information Specialists. 2nd ed. Berkeley, Calif., Alcohol Research Group, Medical Research Institute of San Francisco and University of California, Berkeley, 1991.

Statistics Sources. 19th ed. Detroit, Gale Research Inc., 1996.

7. JOURNAL LISTINGS

The Serials Directory. An International Reference Book. Birmingham, Ebsco Publishing, annual (supplemented by quarterly updates).

Ulrich's International Periodicals Directory, Now Including Irregular Serials & Annuals. New York, R. R. Bowker Co., annual (updated between editions by *Ulrich's Quarterly*).

> See: Subject categories, such as drug abuse and alcoholism, medical sciences, pharmacy and pharmacology, psychology, public health and safety.

8. AUDIOVISUAL PROGRAMS

The Directory of Medical Video Programs. Hawthorne, N.J., Ridge Publishing Co., 1990.

National Library of Medicine Audiovisuals Catalog. Bethesda, Md., National Library of Medicine, 1977-1993, quarterly, with annual cumulations.

> See: *MeSH* terms as noted in Section 1 under *Index Medicus*.

Patient Education Sourcebook. 2v. Saint Louis, Mo., Health Sciences Communications Association, c1985-90.

> See: *MeSH* terms as noted in Section 1 under *Index Medicus*.

9. GUIDES TO UPCOMING MEETINGS

Scientific Meetings. San Diego, Calif., Scientific Meetings Publications, quarterly.

> See: Subject indexes.

> See: Association listing.

World Meetings: Medicine. New York, Macmillan Pub. Co., quarterly.

> See: Keyword index.

> See: Sponsor directory and index.

World Meetings: Outside United States and Canada. New York, Macmillan Pub. Co., quarterly.

See: Keyword index.

See: Sponsor directory and index.

World Meetings: United States and Canada. New York, Macmillan Pub. Co., quarterly.

See: Keyword index.

See: Sponsor directory and index.

10. PROCEEDINGS OF MEETINGS

*Directory of Published Proceedings. Series SEMT. Science/Engineering/Medicine/Technology. White Plains, N.Y., InterDok Corp., v.3, 1967- , monthly, except July-August, with annual cumulations.

*Index to Scientific and Technical Proceedings. Philadelphia, Institute for Scientific Information, 1978-, monthly with semiannual cumulations.

11. SPECIALIZED RESEARCH CENTERS

Medical Research Centres. Harlow, Essex, Longman, biennial.

International Research Centers Directory. Detroit, Gale Research Co., annual.

Research Centers Directory. Detroit, Gale Research Co., annual (updated by *New Research Centers*).

12. SPECIAL LIBRARY COLLECTIONS

Directory of Special Libraries and Information Centers. Detroit, Gale Research Co., annual (updated by *New Special Libraries*).

Index

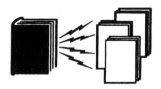 Haworth
DOCUMENT DELIVERY
SERVICE

This valuable service provides a single-article order form for any article from a Haworth journal.

- *Time Saving:* No running around from library to library to find a specific article.
- *Cost Effective:* All costs are kept down to a minimum.
- *Fast Delivery:* Choose from several options, including same-day FAX.
- *No Copyright Hassles:* You will be supplied by the original publisher.
- *Easy Payment:* Choose from several easy payment methods.

Open Accounts Welcome for ...
- Library Interlibrary Loan Departments
- Library Network/Consortia Wishing to Provide Single-Article Services
- Indexing/Abstracting Services with Single Article Provision Services
- Document Provision Brokers and Freelance Information Service Providers

---

MAIL or *FAX* THIS ENTIRE ORDER FORM TO:

Haworth Document Delivery Service
The Haworth Press, Inc.
10 Alice Street
Binghamton, NY 13904-1580

or FAX: 1-800-895-0582
or CALL: 1-800-342-9678
　　　　9am-5pm EST

PLEASE SEND ME PHOTOCOPIES OF THE FOLLOWING SINGLE ARTICLES:
1) Journal Title: _____
　　Vol/Issue/Year: _____ Starting & Ending Pages: _____
　Article Title: _____

2) Journal Title: _____
　　Vol/Issue/Year: _____ Starting & Ending Pages: _____
　Article Title: _____

3) Journal Title: _____
　　Vol/Issue/Year: _____ Starting & Ending Pages: _____
　Article Title: _____

4) Journal Title: _____
　　Vol/Issue/Year: _____ Starting & Ending Pages: _____
　Article Title: _____

(See other side for Costs and Payment Information)

COSTS: Please figure your cost to order quality copies of an article.

1. Set-up charge per article: $8.00

              ($8.00 × number of separate articles) _____

2. Photocopying charge for each article:

              1-10 pages: $1.00 _____

              11-19 pages: $3.00 _____

              20-29 pages: $5.00 _____

              30+ pages: $2.00/10 pages _____

3. Flexicover (optional): $2.00/article _____

4. Postage & Handling: US: $1.00 for the first article/

              $.50 each additional article _____

              Federal Express: $25.00 _____

              Outside US: $2.00 for first article/

              $.50 each additional article _____

5. Same-day FAX service: $.35 per page _____

              GRAND TOTAL: _____

METHOD OF PAYMENT: (please check one)

❑ Check enclosed   ❑ Please ship and bill. PO # _____

          (sorry we can ship and bill to bookstores only! All others must pre-pay)

❑ Charge to my credit card: ❑ Visa; ❑ MasterCard; ❑ Discover;

                 ❑ American Express;

Account Number: _____ Expiration date: _____

Signature: ✗ _____

Name: _____ Institution: _____

Address: _____

_____

City: _____ State: _____ Zip: _____

Phone Number: _____ FAX Number: _____

MAIL or *FAX* THIS ENTIRE ORDER FORM TO:

Haworth Document Delivery Service	**or FAX:** 1-800-895-0582
The Haworth Press, Inc.	**or CALL:** 1-800-342-9678
10 Alice Street	9am-5pm EST)
Binghamton, NY 13904-1580